TRUST YOUR BODY, TRUST YOUR BABY

Peace on earth starts with birth

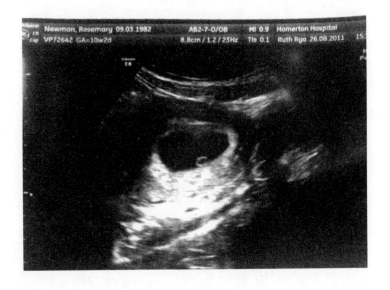

For Luke, Elliott and Arno
My light, my heart and my falling star

TRUST YOUR BODY, TRUST YOUR BABY

How Learning to Listen
Changes Everything

Rosie Newman

Trust Your Body, Trust Your Baby:
How Learning to Listen Changes Everything

First published in Great Britain by Pinter & Martin Ltd 2017

© 2017 Rosie Newman

ISBN 978-1-78066-245-9

British Library Cataloguing-in-Publication Data
A catalogue record for this book is available from the British Library.

Set in Dante

Printed and bound in the EU by TJ International Ltd, Padstow, Cornwall

This book has been printed on paper that is sourced and harvested from sustainable forests and is FSC accredited.

Pinter & Martin Ltd
6 Effra Parade
London SW2 1PS

www.pinterandmartin.com

THE HUMP

You are the sickness that I sought,
The hunger that eats me,
The thirst that cracks my lips.
You are the hump,
That bends me, twists me,
And buckles my back.
You are the swell,
That rolls across the surface,
And churns in the deep.
You are the bump,
That makes me a lump.
Swollen and ripe.
You are juicy and bittersweet,
The fruit of my womb,
The fruit of my labour.

– Rosie Newman

A NOTE FROM THE AUTHOR

I find 'we are having a baby' a funny turn of phrase, because there is no *having* with a baby. There is only *giving* and that is the truth of it. You give your body, you give your time and you give things up. If you're lucky, you will *have* a beautiful, full and significant existence in return. But my perception of 'having' has certainly changed since I became a mother. Having children is more about letting go than holding on. My own family has suffered heavily from the financially crippling decision to live on one income for the early years of our children's lives. But this sacrifice has not gone unrewarded. Our lives have been fundamentally altered in ways we could never have envisioned or chosen and I am so grateful for what we have now.

This book is not a how-to guide. I understand very well that circumstances dictate and restrict our choices, and I know that some of the things I talk about might not even be a remote possibility for some or of interest to others, but that doesn't mean that they should go unsaid. We might as well be honest about the fact that we cannot have it all – at least not all at the same time. Life just isn't like that. We must embrace what we can do rather than dwell on what we cannot. Every parenting journey has its unique trajectory and challenges, be they infertility, multiple births, unplanned caesarean, unplanned formula feeding, same-sex, non-biological or single parenting, disabilities, special needs, infant loss or miscarriage. My point is always the same and it applies to everyone: trust and listening never fail to provide answers to these challenges if we are truly willing to see what is revealed when we open our ears and our hearts to the truth of our nature. This book is in part realistic and in part idealistic. While it is important to be grounded in reality, there is certainly no harm in looking up.

It is my dearest wish that this book might offer something of value to anyone who cares to pick it up. Perhaps not every part of it applies or appeals to every person, but many of the themes and ideas explored are universal. As a breastfeeding peer supporter I have listened to the stories of many, many mothers who felt they had no one else to turn to. They were usually seeking help for specific infant feeding issues, but more often than not, their problems were interlinked with every other aspect of their new life as a mother. It became clear that the real problems lie not in the bodies of mothers and babies, but in the bigger picture that they find themselves a part of. We may all struggle with different issues, but when you talk to lots of people, you start to see patterns emerging. I have written this book with those larger themes in mind.

Lastly, we have a bit of a problem with gendered pronouns in the English language. We don't have a neutral one that can apply to either sex and the word 'they' sounds impersonal to me. I have used 'he' in this book because I had two baby boys and I am writing largely from my own experience, so it felt right to do it that way. When I say he, I just mean 'the baby'.

CONTENTS

SETTING FORTH

The way is not in the sky. The way is in the heart.
– Buddha

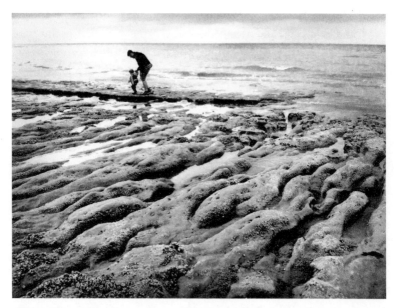

I had no intention of doing things differently. I believed that my ability to multitask would stand me in good stead for successful parenting. Surely a child is a blank slate? How hard could it be? I wanted to breastfeed, but thought that anything beyond six months was a bit weird, and so I had the bottles and steriliser ready. We were given some cloth nappies, but also stocked up on disposables. We bought a cot bed and a Moses basket and spent weeks decorating the nursery. We deliberated endlessly about which buggy was best. We thought 'baby-wearing' was worth a go, but we were happy to use the slings that were handed down to us and didn't give it much thought. I did pregnancy yoga, but didn't bother with hypnobirthing.

I wanted as natural a birth as possible, and even considered a home birth, but fear got the better of me and I opted to go to a birth centre instead – the best of both worlds, or so I thought. I was normal, average, and as it turns out, I was naive.

I didn't read any parenting books while I was pregnant because they all say something different and I didn't know who to believe. We relied mainly on advice from friends and relatives, and when the baby came we tried really hard to follow their suggestions, but more often than not, doing things the 'right' way made everyone miserable and I couldn't understand why it wasn't working. Other people's babies seemed not to mind so much, not to cry so much, not to 'demand' so much. During those bleary-eyed, early days I felt like a total failure, and worse, I felt disconnected from my baby. Everywhere I turned for help, the answers that came made me feel that either he or I, or both of us must be defective and that I wasn't capable of looking after my own child. Most of the books people recommended were either overwhelmingly scientific, or ludicrously simplistic. Many offered cure-all methods that didn't appear to be based on fact, reality or even common sense. I had been so focused on the birth of my baby that I was completely unprepared for what lay beyond. My husband and I were lost in the fog, clinging only to each other and the remote possibility that things would get better.

But in the midst of all that confusion, there were times when I did allow my own judgement to override the impulse to conform and in those moments things seemed a bit better. Little by little, I began to feel the nudge of an idea growing inside me. It felt good and warm and strong. It felt something like confidence, and eventually I couldn't ignore my baby or my instincts any more. The message was coming through loud and clear and whether it's because I'm indulgent, stubborn or just curious, I decided to reject the idea that my baby was faulty and I started to listen. I started to trust – in us.

I realised that for nine months I had known he was coming,

but he knew nothing of me or the outside world before he landed in my arms. However genuine my intentions were, he had no way of knowing unless my actions met with his needs. I began to understand that if I wanted his trust, I would have to earn it. From his perspective, as a creature of pure instinct and emotion, with no capacity for reasoning, if he fell asleep in my arms but woke up alone, then that was a betrayal and a reason to fear. He wanted, needed, expected me to be there for him. What I was being told to do wasn't what he needed and all the love in the world could not undo that fact.

I began to notice that there are people who are quietly doing things differently with their babies. There is a fresh effusion of new ideas emerging from modern science and ancient wisdom and it is permeating the fabric of our culture, chasing away the stagnant whiff of Victorian values – that old miasma that has started to become a bit offensive.

When I focused only on my baby and on my own sense of direction, I could begin to unpick the tangled web of my preconceived ideas and I started to wonder where they had come from in the first place. What followed was the inexorable unravelling of all the knots of anxiety and fear that had had me tightly bound. I gained a new perspective on myself, my family, my society, our history and the whole world around me. I discovered tools that have enabled me to resolve conflicts and to reconcile past traumas. I have learnt to trust. I have learnt to listen. I have learnt to let go. And everything has changed, for the better.

1. STOP THE CLOCK

Time is an illusion.
– Albert Einstein

The time has come. It's baby time. The beginning of the rest of your life. From this point on there is only the time before you had a baby and the time after you had a baby. This is one event that will unfailingly form an indelible punctuation mark in the story of our lives and everything that comes afterwards hinges upon it. Time suddenly seems very significant, but ironically now is a good time to try and let go of clock-watching altogether. We have collectively developed an obsession with timekeeping and it's great for managing busy careers and social lives, but it's worse than useless when it comes to managing babies. Babies can't tell the time and they couldn't care less. The time will drive you crazy and that is a stone-cold fact. So I dare you to experiment with giving up all things horological, because the clock is no longer your friend. If you're not careful, it will become your unforgiving master, and you its willing slave. Concerns about your biological clock may well have been a headache before you became pregnant, but starting from the (precisely recorded) time he or she arrives, you will be encouraged to monitor and control your baby's every move. From his daily feeding and sleeping patterns to his major developmental milestones, from this moment on the clock is king, and there's even an app for it.

And it appears to be everyone else's business to know about your baby's routine as well. Friendly old ladies on the bus, well-meaning shop assistants, even the postman might ask you whether your baby is 'good'. By this they mean can you leave him sleeping alone in his cot for ages without waking up and crying? People are more likely to offer unsolicited advice about how to 'get the baby down' than they are to offer to fix you a snack or hold him while you have a shower. But the majority of questions will come from other mothers who are seeking to compare their own experiences with yours. Exhausted and anxious, we are hoping for a nugget of useful information, and attempting to gauge how our own babies are faring in the ultimate quest for 'normality'. For some reason, it appears that averageness has become the benchmark for success when it comes to babies. Those that don't conform to the centre of the bell curve are likely to be deemed unwell, problematic or just not 'good'.

The dreaded bell curve of normality applies to pregnancy and birth as well. If our babies present in an 'unfavourable' position, or our BMI is 'too high', we won't fall into the golden category of low risk. We will be fast-tracked onto a medicalised birthing pathway and faced with the systematic removal of choices which that entails. There is of course a strict schedule of tests and scans during pregnancy to get the ball rolling, which gets us into the habit of monitoring our progress as we go along. We count the days (hoping the baby doesn't come too early) until his due date finally arrives, at which point we suddenly face a two-week deadline within which to 'deliver'. Beyond this loom the dark cloud of artificial induction and the uncertainty of 'increased risk'. *Tick tock, drip drip*, we're starting to feel the pressure. Targets, timings, centimetres and millilitres, judgements and comparisons are made at every opportunity. You can end up feeling anxious, even when things *do* measure up.

It's hard to pinpoint exactly why it has become like this, but it has a lot to do with the advent of a technological, medicalised approach to birth and childcare. There's no doubt that in many cases, the safety net of Western medicine is reassuring and even life-saving. But for many new mothers, tentatively stepping out onto a totally new path, the language of risk assessment sows a seed of doubt in our minds that can steal the wind from our sails and the temerity that we need to see us through it under our own steam.

Definitions of 'normal' vary all over the world, and one of the biggest challenges of having a baby in a multicultural society is the clash of parenting styles that are in use within it. We are confronted with a baffling array of choices and sometimes it is impossible to get our bearings and connect with our own internal compasses. So in this book, I'm going to try to redress the balance, and talk about why I believe that we know more than we think we do about how to be a mother or a father. I'm officially handing over the torch that has been carried by parents throughout the millennia. Listen to yourself and to your baby, and don't be afraid of what you hear.

Knowledge is your ally in making choices you can believe in. I would like to share all the things I wish I had known before I had a baby. There are some really neat ideas out there – information and ways of doing things – that should have floated to the front and centre of our collective consciousness, but instead they languish in an 'alternative' pigeonhole on the outskirts of our cultural mainframe. Basically, if there's no money to be made from it or it stands in the way of money being made, we just don't hear about it. Some things are so amazing you won't believe that they're not common knowledge. Did you know there is *no significant compositional difference* between infant first formula and so-called 'follow-on' milk? Did you know that young babies have a reflex that allows them to control their bladder and bowel movements? Did you know that carrying a baby upright in a sling helps his core muscles and inner ear to develop, improving his motor skills with every step, squat or sway that you make?

I know what it's like to trawl through books and websites for the really helpful stuff, so I will try not to weigh things down too much with facts and figures. I'm certainly not going to tell you

I have all the answers. This book is not a cure-all, or a how-to manual. I don't believe such a thing exists. Parenting is not about getting it right. It's about getting the right attitude. I'm not an expert on any children other than my own, but I'm fine with that because I rarely find the words of the self-proclaimed childcare 'experts' to be of much help anyway. They often contradict one another, despite the supposedly concrete evidence that proves they are right. Research findings tend to vary depending on who is interpreting them, and the vast majority of research is carried out or funded by people who stand to make money from it. Some things can be said to be irrefutable fact, but much of what is espoused by so-called experts is either conjecture or it cannot be backed up because the research it is based on was either biased or done on too small a scale to be fully representative. The only thing that helped me make sense of the challenges I faced was hearing the experiences of other mothers. It made me realise that the answer to any given question depends entirely on the people involved, not on what others think.

I'll try to put parenting into perspective, globally and historically, and remove it from the narrow scope of medical orthodoxy that often dominates our thinking. Feel free to take only what is helpful to you, and leave the rest. Trusting in yourself starts now, because *Trust Your Body, Trust Your Baby* is about all the things that I hope you will instinctively recognise to be true because they just make sense. If you find ideas in this book that help you feel that you have the right and the ability to decide how you nurture your own family, I will have done what I set out to do. So grab a snack and let's get started!

2. A PREGNANT PAUSE

Everything will be alright in the end.
So if it is not alright, then it is not yet the end.
– The Best Exotic Marigold Hotel

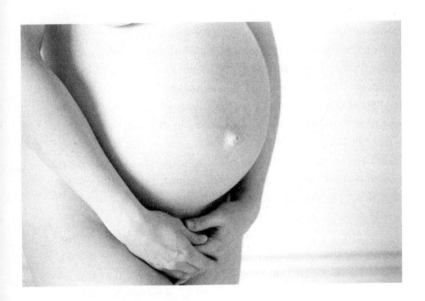

I) BE LIKE WATER

The fundamental lesson that pregnancy offers us is patience. We have to wait. There is no rushing a pregnancy. Things are taken out of our hands and decisions are made on our behalf. We have no choice but to surrender to the process. The baby has a glorious window of 40 weeks where he has total control over his own environment. He builds a protective cocoon around himself and basks in a warm bath of love and serenity. But did I spend those precious nine months reflecting on the importance of patience, on accepting that all things come in their own time and on letting nature take its course? No. For the most part, my first pregnancy was a time spent getting ready for the moment when control would be handed back to me, and I could start making everything fit together again, 'the way it should'.

'For Tibetans, pregnancy can be a highly spiritual time, laden with tradition and ritual. Women are urged to constantly meditate and pray, think positive thoughts, and do good deeds.'[1] In traditional Maori culture too, pregnant women take time to reflect every day with a ritual of breathing deeply at sunrise and sunset. But in most Western cultures, there is no such reverence. Far from being a time of ritual and reflection, pregnancy is a juggling act of all the usual things that life throws at us, plus a few little extras: blood tests, antenatal classes and finding the perfect curtains for the nursery. We pay lip service to the significance of pregnancy, but in reality it's business as usual and we are lucky to be offered a seat on the bus.

We are waiting, but not necessarily patiently, until we can show our baby to the world and mould him into the child of our dreams. Efficiency and goal-orientated thinking may be helpful in the workplace, and they are universally encouraged in capitalist culture, but they are part of a system that is simply *not* compatible with babies. Babies are on slow-time. Any attempt to hurry or 'achieve' anything is stressful beyond belief. Pregnancy is the perfect time to reflect on a change in perspective and a change of pace, and this is probably the single most helpful thing any parent can do to prepare for the arrival of a baby. Learning to let go of outcomes and live in the present moment will not only help with the birth, but all that lies beyond it too.

Before I became pregnant for the first time, I thought that children were the product of their parents: nature and nurture combined. But I had no idea how much *I* would become a product of my child. Looking back, perhaps I was lucky to have been overwhelmed by severe pregnancy sickness (hyperemesis). This condition let me know early on that I was not really in control. It was fair warning that my baby had his own ideas about how things needed to be done. And if reading that just made your heart sink, then fear not. It's actually not a bad thing. Babies have got their priorities straight, and we could learn a lot from them.

They may not be able to speak, but babies are born with the wisdom of the ages. They don't need anyone to agree with them in order to be completely certain about what matters. They are pure instinct, and what they know, they know with every cell of their being. They are built to survive, and everything they do, they do for a good reason. As adults we often feel sure that we must know better. But with all the years of intellectualising that come with growing up, we tend to only grow further from the truth of what makes us happy. Primitive instincts are replaced by logic and reasoning, which may allow us to function in a modern society (and it has certainly helped us to succeed as a species), but we have lost the connection with our primal selves. We no longer feel comfortable in our natural environment, or even in our own skins.

'Three weeks old, warm and gently snoring on my shoulder as I write, you are closer to nature than you will ever be again. With your animal needs and animal cries, moved by a slow primordial spirit that will soon be submerged in the cacophony of thought and language, you belong, it seems to me, more to the biosphere than to the human sphere. Already it feels like years since I saw you, my second daughter, in the scan, your segmented skeleton revealed like an ancient beast uncovered by geologists, buried in the rock of ages.'[2]

It can be hard to imagine what life is like for a baby. I have often heard people saying things like 'What have you got to complain about?' or 'I wish I had your problems', when referring to a crying infant. But pregnancy can provide a glimpse at the experience of being a baby, and believe me, there is plenty to complain about. Being pregnant can make us feel vulnerable in a way that we haven't felt since we were tiny ourselves. We may suddenly want or need our loved ones to look after us, to spare their time for us, to feed us, to hold us. And having to rely on others like this can be frightening, unsettling and unfamiliar. In pregnancy our bodies are changing rapidly, doing new things that we can't control. There are uncomfortable new sensations, extreme hunger, fatigue and hormonal changes. We basically feel a bit like a baby again, and for many of us, it's no picnic.

I was completely immobilised by *hyperemesis gravidarum* (HG) during both my pregnancies and I was often so tired and hungry that all I could do was cry. People told me that I should eat ginger biscuits and get on with it. They thought I was making a bit too much fuss and I was inclined to agree with them. I felt ashamed of the apparent weakness and inadequacy of my body. But after I had my baby I noticed that people often said similar things to me about *him*. They said he was fussy – that he was manipulating me and that it was in his best interests to let him cry, to self-soothe, to get on with it. I wouldn't wish HG on anyone, but if there is a silver lining to be taken from that experience, it is empathy for the helpless and the wisdom to believe that a baby has good reason to cry, even if that reason is not glaringly obvious to me.

Hyperemesis is a serious illness, and it is *not* the same as morning sickness. Many women struggle through it with no extra help because often there simply is none. Some even miscarry or have to abort their babies, because they cannot stop working, or the pregnancy threatens their own life. This often happens quietly, behind closed doors, and because the world can't see what is happening, it effectively doesn't exist. Unfortunately, it is taboo in our culture to talk about a pregnancy 'too early' in case a mother loses the baby. But mothers deserve support during this time, and it is everyone's business to be there for us, whether the baby survives the first trimester or not.

There should be a form of maternity leave available for women who experience severe pregnancy sickness, because many women are unable to work through it. But of course you *are* working when you are pregnant. Just because pregnancy doesn't occupy your hands does not mean that your body isn't working. Not only are you creating an entirely new living being, you are making a large additional organ (the placenta), and 30 per cent more blood than usual. It's amazing to learn that a flash of light in the form of 'radiant zinc fireworks' is emitted at the time of fertilisation.[3] This marks the start of the gathering of life force that is the gestation of a new being. Like the birth of a new star, we are talking about the beginning of energy itself. It can literally feel like a black hole has opened up in the pit of your stomach, mercilessly draining you for months on end. Life and death occupy the same space at the same time. Anne Enright talks about 'the anxiety of reproduction, the oddness of it, and how it feels like dying, pulled inside out'.[4] The very start of life is raw and elemental. It's not always rainbows and butterflies and it deserves recognition.

To be pregnant is a rare opportunity to connect with your primal self – the human animal that we routinely ignore. It can be a time of inward reflection upon the core of things, on what we truly are, where we come from and on what life is all about. But the continuous focus on risk assessment that takes place during pregnancy means that we are not encouraged to look within ourselves for answers. The focus is taken outwards to what we can do to manage the whole process. Depending on our chosen approach, we will either look to medical interventions like epidurals, or to 'alternative' techniques, like hypnobirthing. They may seem like polar opposites, but essentially, whether we choose a medical or an alternative course of intervention, the message is the same: our bodies need help. Many first-time mothers find it impossible to believe that they are even capable of natural childbirth.

But as legendary midwife Ina May Gaskin reminds us, we are the only species to doubt our ability to give birth. Fear and doubt undermines the natural process, and fear of failure becomes self-fulfilling. Believe it or not, one of the most significant revelations of my life came when I was pregnant and quite by chance I saw some footage of a gorilla giving birth. It was captivating. It was clear that she trusted the messages her body was giving her, in a way that I could not even imagine at the time. She looked relaxed and soft as she swayed and shifted. She was rocking, lowing and squatting, and when the baby began to emerge, she reached down and gathered it up into her chest. She held her baby gently and assuredly. It seemed like she just knew what to do and I found it very moving. In fact, it's a moment I will never forget. With no obstetric understanding about what was happening to her, you might think that she would be frightened, stressed or confused. But her instincts told her everything was okay and seeing this provided a moment of clarity for me.

Despite having all the normal reservations about my own body's abilities, the experience of seeing that gorilla giving birth must have made its mark on my unconscious. On some level, it told me that I had no reason to doubt myself and that, if I listened, my body would tell me what to do. As it turned out, childbirth was not the horrifying experience I had heard about from others. Rather, it was the first time in my life that I truly felt my animal self, and it was weirdly enjoyable. I was amazed at the strange noises I made. It felt good, and not just after it was all over, but during the pain and the pushing. Feeling my body taking over felt like a strange combination of both commanding and surrendering to the energy of the universe. For once, my body was in control and not my mind. I have to say that even though my midwife told me to hold my breath and push as hard as I could, I found that I didn't actually have to. My body just kind of did it. Years later, I read the words of Ina May Gaskin and recognised what had happened: I 'let [my] monkey do it'.

There is a lot of debate about the part that anatomy has to play in the pain of childbirth. While it is true that the human pelvis is narrower than a gorilla's, the contractions of the uterine muscles which open the cervix (the source of much of the pain) are experienced by all mammals. The passage of the baby through the human birth canal requires a twist on the way down, but the ligaments of the pelvis soften during pregnancy, and the baby's head is uniquely malleable, which allows it to mould and fit through the gap in all but a small proportion of childbearing women. A normal, healthy human pelvis is *not* a vice. There are rare instances when a baby's head circumference is too big to fit through the pelvis of his mother and a caesarean is necessary, but this is not common enough to explain the difficulty we in the West seem to have in giving birth.

In Mexico, techniques using a *rebozo* cloth are traditionally used to reposition babies, to support mothers during birth and to 'close' their bodies afterwards. Australian Aboriginal midwives use massage to show the baby where to go, and in China they use herbs and acupuncture to great effect. Our bodies are designed to open and close and Western culture is unusual in disbelieving this fact. Our lack of faith in women's bodies becomes a self-fulfilling prophecy because we need to be relaxed for it to happen and fear or anxiety will often prevent this. I'll admit that before I experienced childbirth I was typically sceptical about the whole idea. I'd heard the analogy about trying to push a watermelon through a hole the size of a lemon. But with a 98 per cent success rate of natural deliveries in a career spanning nearly half a century, Gaskin has complete faith in the ability of the human female to deliver human babies. In her words, 'Your body is not a lemon.'

Letting go of fear and taking ownership is the key to a positive birth experience. It's a case of realising that the monster under the bed is not real. It's a bogeyman that we have been fed stories about since we were children. We don't have to be afraid of a shadow in the dark. It is possible to relax, soften and surrender to the process of childbirth without becoming a victim of it. Remember that we are a powerful ally to the forces of nature, but those forces cannot guide us if we are not willing to trust in them. Our birth team needs to be willing to trust in our bodies too. Instructing us to lie back and push against gravity through gritted teeth is just not an efficient way to birth a baby.

While it is important to be realistic about 'natural' childbirth and of course we must take action when it is necessary, our society does not benefit in the long run from the blanket adoption of default settings that override the natural process and effectively prevent it from unfolding. Our feelings about birth directly affect our feelings towards our babies. If we take the approach of fighting against nature from the very beginning, isn't it possible that we risk creating a pattern of conflict in the way that we relate to our children? If we allow ourselves to believe that nature has got it all wrong, and the relationship between our babies and our bodies is flawed – that the shapes don't match – then we leave ourselves vulnerable to the pervasive idea that our children can be faulty too. Unfortunately, this does appear to be rife in our culture. Children are judged 'good' or 'bad' from their very first weeks on earth. We are diagnosing, disciplining and medicating our children at an ever-increasing rate, but the incompatibility lies not between our babies and our bodies. It lies in the foisting of unnatural parameters and expectations on human animals. My own beliefs about where 'good' and 'bad' behaviour originate has been reconfigured since my experience of having children. I have found it liberating to learn to let go a bit, and perhaps our relationships with our babies depend upon us being able to do so.

Though the bamboo forest is dense, water flows through it freely.
– Hsin Hsin Ming

Remember that it is not a weakness to be flexible and yielding. In describing true strength, Bruce Lee advised his student to 'be like water', and how right he was. Water is the source of life itself. It is strong and soft at the same time. It moves around obstacles, teasing and caressing them until they give a little.

And given time, water has the power to cut through mountains. There is strength in conceding and compromising. The more we push for things to be a certain way the more resistance we create. Being flexible, adaptable and respectful of the obstacles that arise means that we can naturally find the right path to move forward.

II) THE ROAD

Taking to the road – by which I mean letting the road take you – changed who I thought I was. The road is messy in the way that real life is messy. It leads us out of denial and into reality, out of theory and into practice, out of caution and into action, out of statistics and into stories – in short, out of our heads and into our hearts.

– Gloria Steinem

It has often been said that the journey of a thousand miles begins with a single step. And in pregnancy, perhaps the first step is to stop. To take a long, deep breath, look around and think about which direction we're heading in. Very often the decision to have a baby is attended by the worry that it may not even happen. But then it does happen, and before we know it, we're out of the gate and heading off down the road towards a distant finish line that shimmers on the horizon. We can vaguely make out that it involves a baby coming out (though exactly how and when is unclear) and it's getting closer every day – it dominates our thoughts. But it's a mirage. *There is no finish line*, and pregnancy is not a means to an end. So let's allow ourselves to take a moment to turn over a couple of stones along the path. The knowledge we gain from exploring a little gives us the confidence to care for our children in the way that feels most natural when the time comes. It might even help us to steer the course when we hit the rough patches along the way.

III) THE RITE OF PASSAGE

Perhaps all this talk of letting go is making you feel a little bit anxious, so let me be clear. It is one thing to become less controlling, and quite another to hand over control to someone else. But that is exactly what is expected of us when we entrust ourselves to the care of the maternity services. Many women are not aware or made aware of their rights in birth and many do not know that we are 'allowed' to say no. Amali Lokugamage is a consultant obstetrician and gynaecologist and she raises an interesting point about the nature of a woman's status during pregnancy:

> '[P]regnancy is a time of great change for a woman's body and mind [...] which I now regard as a rite of passage. Traditionally, rites of passage entail a period of liminality in which the initiate is considered dangerous to society because he or she is living in a transitional realm between social categories that is not officially acknowledged.'[5]

This liminality means that during pregnancy a woman is effectively in limbo between roles. She is no longer a 'maiden', and not yet a mother. Her uncategorised status impairs her authority during the transitional period. She becomes dependent on her caregivers and as such she is potentially vulnerable to domination and bullying. In Western society, our healthcare providers hold a position of power over us during this time.

We are extremely lucky to have free and accessible healthcare in the UK. There is no denying that doctors and nurses work hard to prevent and intercept serious conditions which can threaten the lives of mothers and babies. But pregnancy itself is not an illness. Few doctors and nurses even witness 'natural' or 'mother-led' childbirth before they are put in charge of a woman's maternity care. Even midwives are usually trained in an environment which dictates that the power in the room lies with the obstetric team, rather than the woman giving birth. The level of intervention that is now commonplace means that obstetrical training revolves around administering and monitoring interventions, rather than observing and assisting the progression of childbirth. Healthcare professionals are primed with knowledge of all the potential ways that the process can fail, and therefore view it as little more than a disaster waiting to unfold. Few women would question a professional who deals with childbirth on a day-to-day basis. We assume that obstetricians are experts in birth, when in fact they are experts in pathology. Lokugamage describes her undergraduate training:

> '[Medical] students were required to be involved in 10 normal and 10 abnormal deliveries [...] There was a lot of theoretical groundwork to cover and of course, as potential doctors who were motivated by altruism and/or the fascination of illness-related problem solving, we were more interested in the pathology or disease of childbirth than the normal deliveries [...] natural childbirth is not really part of the main medical focus.'[6]

Lokugamage eventually chose to have her own baby at home, but it was the experience of pregnancy, rather than her medical training which led her to that decision. In fact, no one was more surprised than she when she decided to have a natural birth. Perhaps her insights into the reality of the medical approach made its inaptitude apparent to her when she became pregnant herself. She was glad to know that medical facilities would be available to her, should she need them, but she also knew that she was entitled to make her own decisions about how and when to use them. She went on to have a normal birth at home.

IV) ADD TO BASKET?

There are endless lists of 'must-have' baby products for us to puzzle over. Department stores shrewdly compile them with tick-boxes, so that we can keep track of what we have bought, and see how much we still have left to buy. With every box ticked, we feel we are arming ourselves against the great unknown of parenthood, but what we end up with is a lot of stuff that we will use once and then have to sell on eBay in six months' time. Beware the quicksand that is online shopping. The quaint phrase 'add to basket' implies that we are just picking up a few essentials. But if we could hold what's in that 'basket' in one hand, we probably wouldn't be shopping for it online. 'Add to lorry-load', more like.

This baby-having thing may be a journey into uncharted territory, and it certainly is scary, but loading ourselves up with baggage doesn't help. It only weighs us down. We feel we have to use all of these things, because we paid good money for them, even if it drives us crazy. Better to travel light. We can pick up what we need along the way (and it's rarely what we thought we'd need anyway). The stuffed-to-bursting attics and endless nearly new baby sales across the country attest to that. The list of things I bought, which my babies DID NOT LIKE is *really* long: the Moses basket, the cot, the buggy, the car seat, the doorway bouncer, the 'lounger', the wheelie walker, the bath seat, the play arch, the teddies, the pram toys, the dummies, Sophie le Giraffe... I really could go on. So what *did* they like? Faces, voices, touch. They liked being a part of things – going out and being in the world. Fresh air and people. That's what they liked.

So here goes. A list of stuff I did and didn't find useful:

THINGS YOU **WILL** NEED:

» A mega-stash of **PRE-COOKED MEALS** in the freezer. Ideally not shop-bought ready meals, but healthy, filling, home-made stews, soups, pasta sauces and cottage pies. You'll need fuel after the baby comes and you won't have time to cook, so unless you have someone at home who's going to act as chef for you in the first couple of weeks (or months) after the baby is born, you'll be glad you spent time squirrelling away some nuts.

» A **SLING**. Or two. Or three. Why? We'll get to that in chapter six but for now it suffices to say that babies need to be carried, and you need your arms free. There are lots of different kinds of baby carrier, but don't be daunted. Do some research and talk to others who use them if you can. Be aware that they vary greatly, and be suspicious if they're very cheap. What might seem like a bargain will soon become a total waste of money if it's uncomfortable. Different carriers suit different body types, but many are not particularly well-designed for long periods of use and can be damaging to your back. Equally important is the design from the point of view of the baby's posture. Ideally his bottom should be well supported so he's in a froggy position, knees held in line with his hips, not hanging down like he's wearing a parachute harness. His body should be tucked in high and close, so his face isn't squashed into your chest and there's no risk of suffocation. Check to see if there is a sling library in your local area so you can try a few out and get some advice.

Wrap slings can be tied in a number of ways to suit you and your baby. Watch demos online and practice in advance, so you have some confidence about how to wrap and how to get the baby in and out before the time comes. 'Stretchy' wraps are only useful for newborns. If you want to use a sling for more than a couple of months it's important to use one that doesn't stretch lengthways. I carried my son in a wrap sling until he was 18 months old. I wore it like an item of clothing, leaving it on all day and taking the baby in and out as I went along. I moved on to a buckle-fastening carrier once he was walking more and sleeping less. It was quick and easy to take on and off. Neither of these won me any prizes in the style stakes, but they were extremely practical. There are some really beautiful woven wraps available if you are willing to invest. There is definitely something out there for everyone. You can even wrap carry twins.

» A **CAR SEAT**. You'll need one for taxis even if you don't drive.

» A **BUGGY/PUSHCHAIR/STROLLER/PRAM**. Whatever you call it, I personally felt like a donkey pushing a cart and never got on with it. You don't *have* to get one, and certainly not for the first couple of months (when your baby may find the idea of being strapped into a carriage of any kind abhorrent anyway). There are plenty of places in the world where people do not use buggies and they seem to cope. We didn't use a buggy at all with my second child and I suffered no ill effects. In contrast, my husband developed carpal tunnel syndrome from pushing our first child in a buggy. So make sure you choose one that is light, manoeuvrable and easy to fold. You can't judge a buggy by its rain cover. Good looks can be deceptive. If you wait a couple of months after your baby comes, you can see how your new-mum friends get on and then pick the best one.

» Good **MATERNITY BRAS**. A nursing bra that is not so ugly that it makes you want to cry can be hard to find, especially if you are an 'unusual' size (as quite a lot of us are). Get measured in a store and if they have nothing nice in your size (quite probable), then look online for something decent. Read the reviews, as people will often leave feedback on the fit. Figleaves, Hot Milk and Bravissimo have a wide range. You'll need to do without underwiring for the first few months of breastfeeding, but for long-term breastfeeding, there are some underwired nursing bras out there for the determined shopper.

» **BABY CLOTHES**. Get acquainted with nearly new sales and online swap shops. You can get a shed-load of hardly worn baby clothes for next to nothing. People are desperate to shift the stuff once they're done with it. (If family and friends want to buy you something, ask for a freezer full of lasagne instead.) By all means buy a couple of new items that you really love, but remember that they will all get covered in poo and vomit immediately, so navy blue, khaki or sunshine yellow are the only practical colour choices, otherwise, it's stain remover at the ready, folks. And to really rain on the Babygro parade, remember that all those gorgeous, tiny, innocent-looking garments were probably made by children in a sweatshop thousands of miles away. Sad but true.

» **FOOD FOR THE BABY**. If you breastfeed, you're good to go. Get some breast pads to soak up the inevitable leakage (oh, the damp circle of shame), a feeding pillow and some lanolin nipple cream. If you bottle-feed you'll need a bit of kit, but everything will be available to pick up second-hand. Just clean it thoroughly first.

» **MUSLIN SQUARES**. An incredible amount of fluid is ejected from babies. You'll need a cloth. (Why these are usually white, I will never understand. I dyed ours purple for our second baby).

» **NAPPIES**. Or not (see chapter 8).

» **HELPING HANDS**. Anyone. Just anyone to pass you a wet wipe when you need one.

THINGS YOU **WON'T** NEED:

This is a *really* long list, so I'm going to abbreviate.

» The instruction manuals. Any book that tells you how best to look after your baby and get it to do what it 'should' be doing is a waste of time. I had a friend who followed a well-known baby book word for word. She had a very contented little baby, who happened to have a naturally mild temperament.

But the guidelines about stretching out the feeds caused her to develop mastitis so badly that she stopped breastfeeding altogether. This contributed to her developing postnatal depression. She loved her baby, but something was missing in terms of feeling empowered and connected. Trusting in yourself and your baby is not just for the baby's benefit.

» Just about everything on the nursery checklists that the shops write. Three different kinds of thermometer? Really? A baby-changing table? Uh-uh. Buy things second-hand, if at all. They will probably get poo or vomit on them at some point. And don't even get me started on baby change bags. They're just regular handbags made out of tablecloth fabric with a plastic mat in a 'special pocket'. What a con.

» Baby shampoo. Seriously, you don't need to wash a baby's hair with anything other than water. Coconut oil after a bath is really good for softening cradle cap so you can comb it out. (Coconut oil is also the best moisturiser I have ever used.) My four-year-old still doesn't need shampoo and his hair is glossy and healthy and clean. Another con.

» Lastly, I have to mention the dreaded clock. Despite what baby experts say, you don't actually have to live by the clock. You really don't. As a rule of thumb, a baby is full when he stops drinking and has had enough sleep when he wakes up happy. Given a little time and encouragement, it is something we are perfectly capable of working out for ourselves.

When in doubt, save your money for a holiday. That's something that everyone will need.

3. BELIEVING IN BIRTH

And the end of all our exploring will be to arrive
where we started and know the place for the first time.
– T.S. Eliot

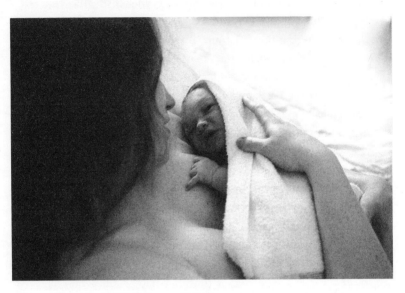

I) SQUATTERS' RIGHTS

Ask an obstetrician the reason why humans have trouble giving birth and the answer will be that we walk on two legs. During the course of our evolution the human pelvis gradually narrowed in order to support our weight and move efficiently when we stood upright. This made the birth canal more restricted, so humans ended up being good at marathon running and disco dancing, but not so good at childbirth. There is also the large human brain to take into account. It is said that human babies are born three months too early because if they weren't, their heads would not fit through the pelvis.[1] The knowledge of this evolutionary twist of fate has cast doubt upon the viability of the whole set-up. The 'obstetric dilemma', as it is known, predicates that we are condemned to fail because of a faulty design feature. But perhaps it is not the *baby's* brain that is the real problem here. Despite the relatively large size of a human baby's head, he will be born before it gets too big and the bones of his skull will not be fused yet, as they are in other ape species, which means they can shift about a bit and squeeze through the gap. Human babies have adapted to the narrowed pelvis. The large prefrontal cortex of the *adult* human brain, however, poses a considerable barrier to successful birth. Our unique ability to analyse and question the mechanics of our own anatomy has created problems where none need exist.

When women are not impeded by doubt, and our movements are not dictated or restricted by our caregivers during labour, we instinctively find solutions. We often get on all fours, kneel, or sometimes squat, returning to postures that resemble those of our ape ancestors, and for good reason. In these upright, forward-leaning positions, the pelvis becomes the most open and yielding that it can possibly be, and gravity helps move the baby down. For hundreds of thousands of years, our ancestors bore children in this way. We did a pretty good job of filling the entire planet with humans, so the system cannot have been so very flawed. But this is not the way we typically birth our babies in a modern obstetric setting. So what changed?

The trend for lying down in labour began among members of the upper classes in Northern Europe around the mid-17th century, supposedly after King Louis XIV watched his mistress give birth like this from behind a curtain. Until this point in history most women would have birthed in the traditional way, by kneeling or squatting on a birthing stool. But wealthy women, who were usually attended by physicians, had access to the latest medical innovations, and these interventions were promoted as a modern and efficient way to give birth. It was a sign of distinction to be attended by doctors, regardless of the outcome, which was largely thought to be in the hands of God anyway. As with many upper-class habits, this approach may have simply filtered down as the right or better way to do things. In a time when birth held high risks for both mother and baby (from infection and any number of complications which could not be predicted or treated at the time), the promise of a safer, more controlled labour must have been more than welcome.

But despite this gradual shift in birth culture, the fact remained that men were excluded from the birthing room in the majority of instances (and still are in many traditional cultures around the world). So during the emergence of obstetrics as a medical discipline, very few doctors (who were always male at that time) were able to witness a straightforward natural birth taking place and this hampered the development of the profession. In 1838, Doctor Hugh L. Hodge of Pennsylvania, USA was so frustrated by this that he argued emphatically for doctors to be at every birth, and launched a campaign to promote the idea that birth was *always* dangerous. He advocated propaganda to make people even more afraid of childbirth than they already were: '[I]f females can be induced to believe that their sufferings will be diminished, or shortened, and their lives and those of their offspring, be safer in the hands of the profession; there will be no further difficulty in establishing the universal practice of.'[2] And it worked.

A culture of difference took root between the midwives, who traditionally handled birth, and the obstetricians, who were moving in on their territory. How different things could have been if a mutual concern for the well-being of mothers and babies had united them. Instead it was a lost opportunity at the dawn of modern maternity care. As midwifery was drawn in under the wing of medicine, midwives found themselves placed beneath obstetricians in the new medical hierarchy. Today they must work within the confines of healthcare systems, which are primarily geared towards treating disease rather than attending birth. It's a square-peg-round-hole kind of situation, because in most cases, women giving birth are not sick. But this has somehow been forgotten. In many places around the world, including in the UK, a tension now exists between what are seen as 'medical' and 'natural' approaches to childbirth. Instead of benefitting from what both professions have to offer, women are often left feeling like we must 'pick a team'.

The story of the persecuted Hungarian midwife Ágnes Geréb illustrates the absurd polarity that persists between midwives and obstetricians even today. Geréb originally trained as an obstetrician, but she was rejected and ridiculed by her colleagues because of her liberal views about how women should be treated during birth. She retrained as a midwife and helped thousands of women deliver their babies safely in their own homes in peace and with dignity. But for a midwife to attend a home birth is illegal in Hungary and in 2010 Geréb was arrested and then imprisoned. One Hungarian mother, Anna Ternovszky, whose home birth Geréb attended, felt compelled by this injustice to take her right to a home birth to the European Court of Human Rights, and she won. This was a landmark case, and the fact that it even had to be fought proves that a woman's right to decide what happens to her body during childbirth still needs to be defended even in an industrialised EU member country like Hungary.

There are countless cases in Western countries of women being coerced, pressurised or even forced against their will into having surgical deliveries, episiotomies and other major medical interventions.[3] In 2013, Kimberly Turbin filed a groundbreaking lawsuit in California, USA against an obstetrician who gave her an unnecessary and unprofessional episiotomy against her will during the birth of her first child. Having had an epidural, she had only pushed twice when her doctor picked up his scissors and decided it was time to take matters into his own hands. He dismissed her request for a discussion about it first, saying, 'What do you mean, "Why?" That's my reason. Listen: I am the expert here.' When Kimberly pleaded, 'But why can't I try?' the doctor answered, '"Why can't I try?" You can go home and do it. You go to Kentucky.'[4] He then cut her perineum 12 times before pulling her baby out.

Turbin suffered from post-traumatic stress disorder following this ordeal and despite contacting the hospital and over 80 lawyers, law firms and non-profit organisations asking for help, nobody would represent her case. Many responded saying that as long as no one died, there was no case to put forward. It is rare for anyone to refute a doctor's authority when it comes to childbirth, and women's rights are therefore effectively wiped off the agenda. But Turbin was unusual in the fact that she had irrefutable evidence because the whole thing was captured on film by her mother. Eventually she had no choice but to represent herself in court and the trial continues. Obstetric medicine protects us from many of the perils of childbirth, but it has created an unexpected new area of risk for women. At best a hyper-medicalised birth can cause unnecessary complications, difficulty with recovery and problems with bonding and breastfeeding. But at worst it can involve outright abuse and lead to post-traumatic stress, postnatal depression and fear of childbirth. Just because nobody dies doesn't mean no harm is done.

But how did it come to be that women accepted being instructed to lie on their backs and have things done to them without consent? And what brought about the change from upright birthing positions to reclining ones? In the time before labour wards, when women usually birthed at home, a doctor would only be called if there was a problem. The mother would be in pain, overwhelmed and exhausted. She would be asked to lie on her back like any sick patient as this would enable the doctor to examine her and carry out procedures, but it immediately places a woman in a subordinate position and it puts the doctor in control. An obstetrician's role was never to observe what was going on, it was always to treat a patient – to do something. This distinction is critical when we try to understand the obstetric tendency towards intervention. The word obstetrics comes from the Latin *obstetrix*, which derives from *obstare*, meaning 'to stand in front of' (from which the word 'obstacle' also comes). The word 'midwife' comes from ancient Middle English, meaning 'with woman'. One word implies power; the other, partnership.

Obstetrics gathered pace as a profession in 17th-century Europe and obstetricians really needed to study the female pelvis in order to understand and document the mechanisms of their science. But their observations of live births were not particularly enlightening, so they turned to the autopsy tables and examined female cadavers. In those days the cause of infection was not understood, and many doctors happily moved between dead and living patients, without ever washing their hands. Between the 17th and 19th centuries, there were astronomically high death rates from puerperal (childbed) fever among women who gave birth in laying-in hospitals, where these autopsies were also being performed. These were places for destitute women with nowhere else to go to have their babies. No one made the connection between the doctors' examinations of the dead and the transferral of diseases to healthy women. It was thought that their 'unclean' souls were the cause of their affliction and not the unclean hands of the doctors. A leading obstetrician and teacher from Philadelphia, Charles Meigs asserted, 'Doctors are gentlemen, and gentlemen's hands are clean.'[5]

There was another unfortunate consequence of the penchant for autopsy examinations among early obstetricians. Ina May Gaskin observes, '[F]ew medical men [of this period] were aware that a living woman's pelvis is very different from that of a dead woman's. The four bones of the pelvis of a living woman are able to flex and move in relation to each other, while the pelvis of a woman who has died is fixed in size and shape.'[6] As a result, medical textbooks and teachings were, for a long time, based on the notion that a baby travels through a fixed ring of bone and navigates past a curved tail bone before he can leave his mother's body.

In fact, the ligaments of the pelvis are doused in a hormone called relaxin during pregnancy, which makes them more stretchy than usual. In instances where a forceps or vacuum extraction would be recommended in a medical setting, midwives might adopt a different approach. It is possible for skilled birth attendants to manually increase the diameter of the lower opening of the pelvis during a difficult labour. 'The technique, called the "pelvic press", involves putting pressure on the upper part of the woman's hips (the upper iliac crest) while she pushes. This pressure pinches her hipbones closer together at the top while opening them a corresponding amount at the bottom, thus freeing the stuck head.'[7] Unlike a medically assisted delivery, this non-invasive technique does not damage the mother's perineum or her faith in her own body.

Another ancient technique that Gaskin is famous for adopting has been named after her. The 'Gaskin Manoeuvre' can be used in the case of shoulder dystocia to free the baby's trapped shoulders. This is a rare situation but one of the most serious complications that can occur during a birth. It involves the shoulders becoming stuck after the head has been born, and can result in asphyxia of the baby. Management in an obstetric setting might involve a major episiotomy and even breaking the baby's collar bone to free it. But Gaskin learnt of this technique on a trip to Guatemala in 1976, where it has been used for centuries. It involves moving the mother on to all fours and arching her back to create additional space for the baby's shoulders to move through.

It may have become standard practice for us to lie on our backs for birth, but it is important to remember that it really doesn't help at all. It is so much harder to push a baby uphill, through a compacted pelvis, with your tail bone restricting the opening. Lying down can also constrict the vena cava, a major artery which supplies oxygen to the uterus and placenta. This all contributes to more pain, more distressed babies and the transformation of a difficult process into a torturous one. Many obstetricians have failed to see the connection and have concluded that women's bodies are fundamentally flawed and in need of assistance. And we have believed it too.

For such a simple idea, the Gaskin Manoeuvre has an astonishing success rate. Out of 1,750 births that took place between 1970 and 1991 at The Farm Midwifery Center in Tennessee where Gaskin worked, 35 births were complicated with shoulder dystocia. Three were managed in the traditional way, before Gaskin learnt the technique, and resulted in birth injuries, as is typically the case in normal obstetric practice. Of the remaining 32 incidences that occurred after she learnt it, and in which it was used, none resulted in any form of morbidity or mortality for mother or baby.[8] A key factor in this is that women labouring on The Farm did not have epidurals, and thus were able to change position when the need arose. Many of the medical interventions that are commonplace today, such as anaesthesia, can restrict labouring women's movements and often have unforeseen implications further down the line.

> 'By medicalising birth, i.e. separating a woman from her own environment and surrounding her with strange machines to do strange things to her in an effort to assist her, the woman's state of mind and body is so altered that her way of carrying through this intimate act must also be altered and the state of the baby born must equally be altered. The result is that it is no longer possible to know what births would have been like before these manipulations. Most health care providers no longer know what "non-medicalised" birth is. The entire modern obstetric and neonatological literature is essentially based on observations of "medicalised" birth.'[9]

The wave of medicalisation that took hold of childbirth in the 20th century propelled it out of the home and into the bright lights of the hospital, and the notion that medical care should supplement midwifery was all but lost. Women were often cared for by doctors and nurses rather than midwives, and midwifery itself became medicalised to a new degree. Even in modern midwife-led birth centres, where women are cared for in a way that upholds the ideal of 'normality in birth', decisions must pass through a fine filter of risk assessment, which is dictated by the healthcare system. This affects every decision made and essentially treats women as statistics rather than individuals.

In this day and age one might hope that we would all benefit from everything that obstetrics and midwifery have to offer. It is fair to say that most current obstetric practice has learnt from the mistakes of the past, and some obstetricians have even become advocates for a hands-off approach to birth, but the experience of the vast majority of women today is still of being dictated to by medical professionals. And the decisions that are made on our behalf are not necessarily the ones we would make if we were offered access to our full range of options. Most women who follow the normal care pathway are not aware that in an attempt to mitigate perceived or potential risks, care providers actually put us at risk of a cascade of interventions, which is a self-fulfilling failure to progress, and is primarily due to interference. Although the medical approach gives everyone the illusion of control, it is proven that higher levels of intervention do not necessarily equate to better outcomes for mothers and babies.

In Sweden, a midwife-centred model of care is the norm. There is access to good medical care in the event of a complication, but the rate of interventions is low and the infant and maternal mortality rates are among the lowest in the world as well. 'Overall, it is the safest place in the world to become a mother.'[10] But in the USA, where an obstetric-led approach is considered normal, the outcomes are nowhere near as good. The US ranks 42nd in neonatal mortality rates worldwide.[11] Among the nine industrialised countries with over 300,000 births per year, the US maternal mortality rate is the highest, three times higher than Canada, the UK or Japan.[12] Astonishingly, in the UK we are edging ever closer to an American model of healthcare, which is dominated by private interests, insurance companies and the accompanying quagmire of risk assessment and litigation avoidance. This poses a direct threat to childbearing women in this country.

A study carried out in Iceland between 2005 and 2009 compared the outcomes of 307 home births with 921 hospital births among 'low-risk' women. They found that the rate of induction, epidural, postpartum haemorrhage and neonatal ICU admission was significantly lower when the woman laboured at home. There were also lower rates of caesarean and anal sphincter injury among the home birth group.[13] This is impressive evidence to support the assertion that home birth is as safe, if not safer than hospital birth among low-risk women. But further to this, a 2015 study carried out in the UK included 'high-risk' women. They found that 'planned home birth was associated with a significantly lower risk of intrapartum interventions and adverse maternal outcomes requiring obstetric care [...] and a significantly higher probability of straightforward vaginal birth'.[14] Furthermore, 'babies of "higher risk" women who plan birth in an obstetric unit appear more likely to be admitted to neonatal care than those whose mothers plan birth at home'.[15] It is not clear whether this was because the babies born in hospital were more likely to be unwell after birth, or just more likely to be put into intensive care as a precaution, but either way, the separation involved in admission to NICU has a significant impact on bonding and breastfeeding outcomes, and therefore carries its own risks.

Doctors and midwives today have the tools to help us safely navigate many of the potential pitfalls of having babies, but you don't call a plumber to run you a bath. Some things we need help with, and others we do not. Birth attendants are at their very best when they let us be their guide, responding to rather than managing the process as it unfolds. It is estimated that if pregnant women are well prepared and cared for, only 10 per cent will need any kind of intervention at all during birth.[16] Obstetric gynaecologist Ricardo Herbert Jones describes the responsibility that caregivers have to the women they support as follows:

'Childbirth is a crossroad. You can help the woman make a fantastic transformative journey in her life… She can understand that since she can surpass all these barriers of pain and fear and accomplish her goal, she can do anything. But at the same time, if we do not respect this woman, and we don't give her dignity during her childbirth we could put her in a situation of depression, and create the idea that her birth is an example of her inferiority, her incapacity, her defectiveness.'[17]

II) INA MAY GASKIN'S SPHINCTER LAW

The 'Three Ps' of obstetrics are the Passenger (baby), the Passage (pelvis) and the Powers (contractions). This suggests that the outcome is predetermined, and can be calculated according to the values of these variables. By this logic, if labour stalls, it is because the baby is too big, the pelvis is too small or the contractions are too weak. But this simplistic view does not take into account the influence of the autonomic nervous system on a woman's physiology. Ina May Gaskin likens the cervix to the sphincter – a ring of muscle that opens and closes. If you apply the Sphincter Law to the equation, labour actually stalls because the external conditions are incorrect.

The cervix behaves in a similar way to the sphincter. Just like the muscles that control our bowel and bladder, the cervix is shy: it will only open up when we are feeling safe and calm. This is a survival necessity which enables our bodies to abandon non-essential functions during a life-or-death event. It is an autonomic response and is built into our primitive nervous system. It is well documented that if an animal in labour feels threatened its body will automatically close up shop until the danger passes. The same rule applies to the human animal. Disruptions, changes of location and conversations about potential problems and risks can have this effect. A shift-change involving a new doctor or midwife is a common enough occurrence, but it registers in our unconscious as a disturbance, ringing alarm bells and calling for vigilance. This is enough to shut things down. All too often the medical response to a stalled labour involves a dose of synthetic oxytocin to get things going again when what may actually be needed is reassurance, patience, calm and quiet.

It is not just fear of birth or an imminent threat that can halt labour. Many women who have strong faith in birth find that when the time comes something in their unconscious mind is obstructing the process. Relationship issues, financial worries or fears for the future can all affect how we feel about labour. A thoughtful, supportive and preferably familiar birth partner can help us to realise and work through our fears. Perhaps this is why doulas and private midwives are becoming increasingly popular. When you get to know someone during your pregnancy you can trust them with your emotional needs during birth.

Doulas can often help us unpack our emotional baggage before birth and can support us with calming techniques that are built up during pregnancy. This is a luxury that we have to pay for, but there is a lot to be said for the power of visualisation and anyone can do that for free. Many hypnobirthing advocates suggest imagining a flower unfurling, which can certainly be helpful, but remember, a vagina is not a fragile flower. It is a specifically adapted organ with amazing capabilities. Its primary function is to do the job of getting babies out, and it is fully qualified. Women's bodies have been known to push out babies while in a coma. Childbirth is not something we really need to think about. In fact, the less we think the better. Our bodies can do it. In *Birth Matters*, Gaskin says:

> 'I remember showing a first-time mother with my hands how much her body would open during birth, and she surprised me by opening more […] than I had ever seen before in a first-time mother […] When I later asked her how she had accomplished this feat […] she told me that with every push, she had held the image in her mind of how huge she was going to get.'[18]

The cervix likes peace and privacy to operate well. Just like the sphincters, it is capable of closing as well as opening, which is why relaxation is so important. Any form of stress, conscious or unconscious, can have an arresting effect on labour. Birth attendants who nurture you and put you at ease are essential. Laughter is also great for helping your cervix to open. Ever done a little wee while you were laughing? It's hard to stay tense during a good chuckle. You may not feel like laughing once you get to active labour, but early on it helps with relaxation and dilation. Ina May Gaskin confirms this in her book *Birth Matters* when she says, 'laughter helps to open sphincters and to keep them open'.[19] She also swears by the power of the kiss. Soft, open-mouth kissing is a sure-fire way to open the cervix; in fact, anything that relaxes the facial muscles seems to have a corresponding effect on the cervix and vagina. A rush of blood is just the ticket for allowing the tissues to swell and stretch, ready for the baby to pass through. It's also a lovely way to make partners feel they are a welcome and necessary part of the birth process and it can strengthen the bonding experience for both parents.

III) ECSTATIC BIRTH

Birth is movement. Birth is a dance!
– Sheila Kitzinger

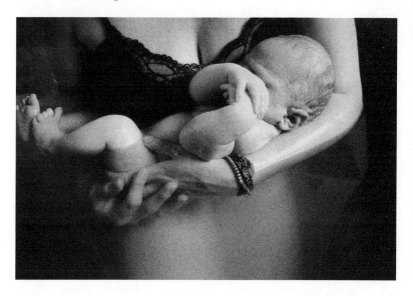

Pleasure is certainly not something most people immediately associate with birth. The idea of kissing your partner through the surges might sound like the last thing you would want to do, and I'm not about to tell you it doesn't hurt. But many women really do find birth to be a highly sensual and even pleasurable experience. Birth stories are always a mixed bag of pleasure and pain. A heady mix of agony and ecstasy. But what we usually hear is that the ecstatic part was the eventual arrival of the baby, not the labour itself. A hysterical media shouts at us from every corner, and we are bullied into believing that birth is horrific. But there is another side to the story and we all need to hear about it.

Ecstatic (or sometimes even orgasmic) birth is a tantalising phenomenon, which many people scoff at and most women do not even dare to hope for. It is a reality, but the conditions that allow it to happen are extremely hard to replicate in a clinical setting. In the same way that pleasant sexual experiences require comfort, dignity and privacy, so too does the act of childbirth. Dr Marsden Wagner was director of Women's and Children's Health for the World Health Organization from 1992 until 1998, and this is how he describes the appropriate environment for birth to take place. 'It's got to be like it is when you make love with someone. It's got to be safe and secure and uninterrupted. And that is how you have an orgasmic birth. Because birth is sexual.'[20]

It's no coincidence that so many women go into labour in the early hours of the morning, when they are rested, warm, relaxed and comfortable. In fact, melatonin (the sleep hormone) plays a key role in creating uterine contractions, when combined with oxytocin.[21] But these conditions are lost the moment we change the setting to one which is generally considered 'safe' and 'correct' for the birth to actually happen:

'In nature, when a laboring animal feels threatened or disturbed, the stress hormone catecholamine shuts down labor. Similarly, when a laboring woman does not feel safe or protected or when the progress of her normal labor is altered, catecholamine levels rise and labor slows down or stops.'[22]

It is little wonder that the moment we intervene, the progress of labour is altered and the potential for it to be pleasurable is undermined. Dr Sarah Buckley believes strongly that women are missing an opportunity for a pleasurable experience when we enter the conventional obstetric setting. As she says, '[T]he ecstatic hormones that a mother produces during labour and birth are almost identical to the ecstatic hormones [beta-endorphin and oxytocin] that the mother will produce during the sexual act. In other words, having a baby has a lot in common with making a baby.'[23]

The first birth Ina May Gaskin ever witnessed was an ecstatic one. Having suffered the trauma of a typical 1970s American hospital birth herself, the experience of seeing a woman exalting in labour was mind-blowing and altered her perspective for ever. 'You're giving birth. Your body's in the process of unfolding and opening. Powerful hormones are released in you that not only make your labour much more efficient, they can take it out of the pain category altogether and put you into that pleasure sphere.'[24] She surveyed 151 women in her village, to see how many, if any, had found birth pleasurable. To her amazement, it turned out that 21 per cent had actually experienced orgasm at some time during labour and birth. But how many women would be bold enough to talk about it unless directly asked? It's not that it's so unlikely, it's just unlikely that you'll ever hear about it.

As it turns out, adrenaline and noradrenaline, which are released in the climax of natural birth, are also released during orgasm. The process that puts a baby inside a woman is connected to the process that gets it out of her. During the latter stage of labour (in the absence of medically administered synthetic hormones), the 'love hormones' beta-endorphin and oxytocin, which have been flooding the body and allowing the cervix to open, are suddenly boosted and coupled with a surge of adrenaline. At this point a woman in labour may feel the irresistible urge to push and release her baby. This climax is often characterised by a change in posture and temperament. Women may become more aggressive and louder. They may fling their heads back, shift forward or stand up. This is all part of the body's way of harnessing gravity to release the baby. In an obstetric ward (but sometimes even in a midwife-led unit), we are typically directed to lie back, tuck in our chins, hold our breath, resist the urge to vocalise and push like hell. Trusting in the authority of our caregivers, rather than in our own instincts, we dutifully oblige.

IV) THE FORCE IS STRONG

Many women describe how they push for hours, sometimes with little effect, during the second stage of labour. For others it is over in a matter of minutes, and every expectant mother wonders which side of the fence she will fall on when her time comes. No matter how long the second stage takes, it has been proven that outcomes are better when we are in charge of our own bodies. Directed pushing (when mothers are told what to do) has been shown to have significant adverse effects including foetal hypoxia (deprivation of oxygen to the baby)[25] and Valsalva-style pushing (prolonged pushes with the breath held) has been found to increase foetal heart rate abnormalities when compared with spontaneous 'mini-pushes'.[26] Perineal trauma also increases when women are directed in bearing down[27] and although the World Health Organization advocated the removal of directed pushing from practice internationally in 2003, it remains resolutely commonplace.

Some midwives may argue that the women they care for need help to know how and when to push, and this may well be true given the circumstances. We all know that epidurals can make pushing more difficult because women cannot feel what they are doing. But an emotional block like fear, doubt or confusion can cause a 'failure to progress' through the second stage too. I expected a fight on my hands when it came to pushing my baby out. I thought that I would have to overcome this 'problem' with sheer grit and determination, but as it turned out, it would have been a fight to stop it. The Ferguson reflex causes an irresistible urge to push and is caused by pressure on the perineal muscles. But there is a dramatic phenomenon known as the foetus ejection reflex, which involves very little active pushing by the mother and occurs quickly and spontaneously. It is so rarely seen that its definition sparks debate among birth experts. Like so many of nature's wonders, if it exists, a foetus ejection reflex is an elusive and mysterious thing. Bright lights and loud voices can scare it away.

Home birth advocate, psychologist, nurse and midwife Marianne Littlejohn says that the foetus ejection reflex is rarely seen in hospitals by midwives and doctors. 'It is disturbed by vaginal examinations, fundal pressure, masculinization of the birth environment, electronic monitoring equipment, cameras, even eye contact.'[28] She goes on to describe her experience of seeing it happen:

'The fetus ejection reflex is not a second stage of labour and is usually preceded by a pause where the mother may stop contractions and sleep for several hours or a mother may doze between contractions [...] When a mother is breathing deeply in between contractions and is resting and calm, babies keep their tone and do just fine. The onset of a fetus ejection reflex may seem sudden and the baby is born after three to four expulsive efforts.'[29]

The question of whether internal examinations are helpful is a contentious issue. We want to know how things are progressing, but the procedure can introduce a risk of infection, the results can be misleading, and whatever the midwife discovers, there can be a temptation to 'do something about it'. It is a fine line between assistance and interference when it comes to helping labour progress. One example of where an examination might cause a problem is in the case of an anterior cervical lip. This is when the cervix is not quite dilated yet. Many women start to feel the urge to push before the lip has fully receded, but if the lip is detected, she will be advised not to. 'At some point in labour almost every woman will have an anterior lip because this is the last part of the cervix to be pulled up over the baby's head. Whether this lip is detected depends on whether/when a vaginal examination is performed.'[30] In the following account, midwife Rachel Reed describes a typical scenario following the detection of a lip:

'The woman is told to stop pushing because she is not fully dilated and will damage herself. Her body is lying to her – she is not ready to push. The woman becomes confused and frightened. She is unable to stop pushing and fights her body creating more pain. Because she is unable to stop pushing she may be advised to have an epidural. An epidural is inserted along with all the accompanying machines and monitoring. Later, another vaginal examination finds that the cervix has fully dilated and now she is coached to push. The end of the story is usually an instrumental birth (ventouse or forceps) for an epidural-related problem – fetal distress caused by directed pushing; "failure to progress"; baby malpositioned due to supine position and reduced pelvic tone. The message the woman takes from her birth is that her body failed her, when in fact it was the midwife/system that failed her.'[31]

It is clear that even with the best intentions, birth attendants can obstruct the course of labour without realising it. Women are left wondering who they can trust. Trust is the essential ingredient in any birthing environment, but it seems like it is pretty hard to come by these days. Most of us would feel anxious trying out a new hairdresser, and yet we are expected to entrust our flesh and blood to strangers and without question. We are compelled to believe that trusting in ourselves is risky, but that is exactly what we need to do. World-renowned obstetrician Michel Odent believes that women *can* be trusted to birth naturally – so much so that he does not believe that his own presence in the room is particularly helpful. He describes the circumstances that make the foetal ejection reflex possible as follows:

'A cultural misunderstanding of birth physiology is the main reason why the birth of the baby is usually preceded by a second stage, which may be presented as a disruption of the fetus ejection reflex. All events that are dependent on the release of oxytocin (particularly childbirth, intercourse and lactation) are highly influenced by environmental factors [...] The passage towards the fetus ejection reflex is inhibited by any interference with the state of privacy. It does not occur if there is a birth attendant who behaves like a "coach", or an observer, or a helper, or a guide, or a "support person". It can be inhibited by vaginal exams, by eye-to-eye contact, or by the imposition of a change of environment. It does not occur if the intellect of the labouring woman is stimulated by rational language ("Now you are at complete dilation; you must push") [...] the true role of the midwife is to protect an environment that makes the ejection reflex possible. The point is to keep in mind the basic needs of labouring women. The point is to reconcile the need for privacy and the need to feel secure.'[32]

Unlike the Ferguson reflex, 'a real fetus ejection reflex can occur long before the descent of the presenting part, or long after. It can start before complete dilation, or after. Usually it does not occur at all because the prerequisite is complete privacy [...] I cannot remember one case of an authentic reflex in the presence of the baby's father.'[33]

This level of privacy may not be possible or even desirable for many of us, especially now that fathers play such an important supportive role during childbirth. Sharing in the experience offers couples a unique bonding opportunity that can forge a strong connection between them and their baby. But nevertheless, Odent's points suggest that birth attendants should always be mindful to promote a sense of privacy and dignity, no matter what setting they are working in. The conditions he describes that encourage a foetus ejection reflex point towards what is truly appropriate for a birthing environment. Bright lights, loud noises, the comings and goings of strangers and a loss of autonomy can prevent labour from progressing normally. All too often these are the very things to which we subject ourselves in pursuit of safety and control. It's not that our bodies don't work properly, we just can't birth in a state of primal fear.

V) MAKING WAVES

We now know that proteins originating in the foetus's lungs will naturally trigger labour to start, so it is the baby who lets his mother's body know when he is ready to be birthed and not the other way around.[34] It has been scientifically proven that he is steering the ship, so let's not kid ourselves that this has anything to do with us. In most cases, it's not our call to make. Sometimes it's best to just keep the faith and wait for our babies to cook. Doctors can make babies come out, but they cannot make them *ready* to come out.

There is also some debate about where the lines should be drawn around what full-term pregnancy even means. In the UK, the NHS currently works on the basis that anything between 37 and 40 weeks gestation is full term.[35] But in America, the guidelines were changed in 2013, because of concerns that caesareans were being carried out too early. The American College of Obstetricians and Gynecologists now defines full-term pregnancy as between 39 and 41 weeks.[36] Everyone seems to be in agreement that by 42 weeks a baby needs to come out, but women are likely to be asked whether they would like to be induced well before that time. Rebecca Dekker, founder of Evidence Based Birth, says, '[T]here is a normal range of time in which most women give birth. About half of all women will go into labor on their own by 40 weeks and 5 days (for first-time mothers) or 40 weeks and 3 days (for mothers who have given birth before) [...] The other half will not.'[37] So there's actually nothing wrong with going overdue. In fact, it's normal. The chance of stillbirth does increase slightly at 42 weeks,[38] but it is still only a 0.1 per cent chance. In order to make an informed decision, we need to compare that to the risks involved with having an artificial induction. These include hyperstimulation of the uterus (in which the uterus contracts too frequently, decreasing blood flow to the baby), the use of extra interventions, such as continuous foetal monitoring, the need for additional pain relief and a failed induction leading to a caesarean section.[39] This is known as the 'cascade of interventions'.

The cascade of interventions is now such a common chain of events that it is almost the new normal for birth. An induction often leads to an epidural, which may then lead to an assisted delivery or a caesarean. These procedures lead to a longer recovery, emotional trauma, lower rates of successful breastfeeding, higher chances of suffering from postnatal depression[40] and sometimes the baby requires special care after birth as a result. Often women are not made aware that by having artificial hormonal treatments to speed up labour, we are more likely to need an epidural, because the contractions will be stronger and more prolonged. We are unlikely to be told that we won't benefit from the calming effect of natural oxytocin, because this is blocked by the artificial one. Interventions are no doubt intended to help us, but the result is often counterproductive.

Here is a list of natural induction techniques that may be worth trying before a medical one:

» Long **WALKS** can help to clear the mind and move the baby down, as does bobbing about on a birthing ball and belly dancing. If you fancy a good bit of bogling, then why the hell not.

» **MAKE LOVE**. Yes, we've all heard this one before. Apparently, it's not just something that someone made up to aid the plight of dejected fathers-to-be. Semen contains prostaglandin, which helps stimulate the cervix to ripen. Nipple and clitoral stimulation releases oxytocin, which helps too. You may or may not be in the mood, but I think we can all agree it's better than a drip in your arm.

» **ACUPUNCTURE**, **ACUPRESSURE**, **SHiATSU** and **REFLEX-OLOGY** can all yield excellent results.
» **LAUGHTER**. Yep. All the good feelings. There's not much that laughter isn't good for. With the possible exception of a full bladder of course.
» Drinking **RASPBERRY LEAF TEA** from 37 weeks onwards may help soften the cervix.

If you go past 42 weeks and feel concerned about it, you can opt for daily monitoring and a stretch and sweep from a midwife. If a chemical induction is necessary, you might be offered an internal pessary rather than an IV drip, which means you can stay mobile. It can be a slow process though, and it is sometimes possible to have an initial dose, and then request more time to see if this is effective, before proceeding with anything further.

Sometimes circumstances will conspire against a natural birth, but the vast majority of cases need not involve obstetric manipulation. In 1997, the Albany Midwifery Practice (AMP) was opened in an area of deprivation and ethnic diversity in south-east London, England. The AMP offered women a continuity-based, midwife-led model of care unlike anything that was available locally on the NHS. This meant that during their antenatal care, mothers could get to know a midwife who would then almost certainly be present for the birth of the baby and who would also then care for the mother and her baby afterwards. The AMP had an 80 per cent success rate for spontaneous vaginal birth. They had the highest home birth rate in the country at 43 per cent (compared to 11 per cent nationally) and a very low induction rate (5 vs. 20 per cent nationally).[41] Their caesarean rate was 16 per cent (compared to the 23.5 per cent national average in 2007) and a forceps/ventouse rate of 3 per cent (compared to the national average of 11.1 per cent in 2007).[42]

Continuity of carer has been shown to have significant benefits for mothers and babies including fewer interventions during birth and a significant decrease in preterm births.[43] So getting to know your midwife improves clinical outcomes as well as experiential ones. But in a risk-management climate, the Albany Midwifery Practice came under scrutiny and was closed down in 2007 by the healthcare trust within which it was operating. In a statement, King's College Hospital acknowledged 'the excellent relationships formed between the Albany midwives and their expectant mothers', but said that an investigation showed 'serious shortcomings in terms of non-compliance with Trust policies and risk management'.[44] Instead of working with the midwives to address or resolve those issues, the Albany Practice was shut down.

VI) CUTTING TO THE QUICK

The AMP's statistics were in line with what the World Health Organization (WHO) has found to be the optimal threshold for safe practice in terms of intervention. In 1985, WHO collected and analysed data from all over the world and concluded that caesarean rates should be between 10 and 15 per cent in order to prevent deaths. Anything above that, and in developed countries the number of women dying actually starts going up. The operating theatre might seem like a safe, controlled environment, but a caesarean is major abdominal surgery and things can go wrong. If a caesarean is not essential, then the chances of unnecessary loss of life increase. We often focus on the safety of the baby, but the death of a mother is also a tragedy. Mothers leave behind families, and if the baby survives, a child who will never know their mother. While surgical techniques are improving all the time, a caesarean is not an easy option and recovery can be gruelling. It can also have a detrimental impact on the breastfeeding relationship. Babies whose mothers receive epidurals and/or systemic opioids during labour exhibit reduced breast-seeking and breastfeeding behaviours, and medical interventions generally decrease the likelihood of establishing breastfeeding.[45] It is also financially expensive and I would argue that it is improvident in terms of resources and clinical waste to deliver babies surgically without just cause. We have sleepwalked into a strange situation wherein caesarean birth is not considered extreme, but unmedicalised birth is.

When medical resources are available, but do not predominate, safe natural birth can become 'normal' again. Ina May Gaskin's track record for facilitating natural births with positive outcomes is a testament to the power of a positive birth culture. Working within her small community on The Farm in Tennessee, she and her partners managed to deliver 2,028 babies between 1970 and 2000 with a caesarean rate of just 1.4 per cent and no maternal mortalities. Of those births, 44.7 per cent were first-time mothers, and the figure includes breech and twin births.[46] As the rest of the US was opting for more and more surgical deliveries, the midwives on The Farm managed to remain unswayed. They honed a traditional set of skills which were becoming so rare that women were willing to travel hundreds of miles in order to have their babies there.

The crucial factor that set the community at The Farm apart from the rest of the United States, and allowed them to develop their own birth culture, was their relative isolation. They set out to live as natural a lifestyle as possible. They grew their own food, walked, swam in a lake and cooperated to build their own homes. The women there had all heard first-hand accounts from their friends of successful natural births. Many had even helped out or witnessed them. They had no reason to doubt any of it, and when it was their turn, they knew and trusted their midwives. *Spiritual Midwifery* by Ina May Gaskin contains a collection of birth stories written by women who gave birth at The Farm. It is a rare glimpse at the potential for women to birth naturally, given the right circumstances. One account is particularly poignant, because it was written by a nurse who describes the difference between a normal hospital environment, and her own birth experience on The Farm:

'The [Farm] midwives had safely seen me and my baby through the passage; I had experienced a change in consciousness, a normal, natural, spiritual birth [...] A couple of years later, while in nursing school, I recognized the tremendous difference between my birth experience and that of most women. In my nursing training I saw fetal monitors being used instead of the provision of sufficient nursing staff. I watched hospitals risk the lives of women and their unborn infants with unnecessary drugs and major surgery instead of conscious human attention, patience and skill. In one hospital where I trained, I watched doctors put needles into the spines of young women for epidurals while loudly discussing their vacation and their new boat. I felt so fortunate not to have had a hospital birth. Instead of having my fears increased by impending medical interventions, my fears were lessened by my midwives. Instead of relinquishing control over my labour and birth to hospital staff, I was empowered to birth without drugs or interventions. Birth is a spiritual experience that is unsurpassed in a lifetime, an experience that each woman deserves in a safe and comfortable setting and with a provider whose goal is a safe passage, a new beginning, and the avoidance of unnecessary interventions.'[47]

Rapid advances in surgical technique and infection control has meant that caesarean rates have increased dramatically all over the world. The NHS Institute for Innovation and Improvement website states that in the UK they went from 12 per cent in 1990 to 24 per cent in 2008 with no improvement in outcomes for the baby (risk to the baby is the primary reason for caesarean deliveries in the first place). This is really significant because caesareans are now being done as routine risk *avoidance* procedures, and are not necessarily essential or life-saving. Obstetricians are honing their scalpel skills, rather than their birthing skills and our belief in birth is being eroded at an alarming rate.

It's fair to say that most women would avoid a surgeon's knife if possible. But the experience or expectation of vaginal birth as unbearably painful, unpredictable and undignified means that many women will choose an elective caesarean over a vaginal birth because they gain a sense of control in doing so. Feeling that we have control of our birth experience is of the utmost importance for it to be a positive one. And with surgical techniques improving all the time, more and more women can expect a satisfactory outcome, but there is a danger that a significant set of risk factors (which go beyond the safety of the surgery itself) are ignored or not made clear to women before they elect. First-time caesareans are generally straightforward operations, but the scars that they leave behind mean that any subsequent pregnancy and caesarean carries a greater risk of complications. It becomes increasingly difficult to separate layers of tissues and organs that have fused together during healing. Sometimes the placenta will be attached to the scar tissue and unable to break away. Having had a caesarean, a woman is statistically more likely to have another one, and of course, most women do have more than one baby. Caesareans save lives and they are a blessing, but perhaps we are sometimes at risk of turning this blessing into a curse.

Caesareans carry the following risks for the mother (the likelihood of which increase with every subsequent caesarean delivery):

» Increase in haemorrhages requiring transfusion
» Hysterectomy for uncontrollable haemorrhage
» Accidental cutting of the bowel, potentially leading to peritonitis, colostomy or death
» Accidental cutting of the uterine artery
» Surgical trauma to bladder and ureters
» Increased postpartum infection, scar breakdown
» Scar pain/numbness
» Long-term severe back pain following epidural block

» Increased pulmonary embolism
» Anaesthesia problems, including paralysis and death
» Post-traumatic stress disorder and postnatal depression

And there are also the following risks involved for the baby:

» Accidental foetal laceration
» Respiratory distress, a major cause of neonatal mortality
» Accidental prematurity because the caesarean was performed too early
» Difficulty establishing breastfeeding[48]

VII) LITTLE WONDERS

It is clear that a caesarean poses more immediate risk to the mother than it does to the child, but there is a new area of science, which is starting to explore a phenomenon that has the potential to affect every single baby born by caesarean for his entire life.

The World Health Organization says that non-communicable diseases like cancer, asthma, cardiovascular disease and diabetes now account for around 60 per cent of all deaths. These diseases are typically triggered by the inappropriate functioning or failure of the immune system, which either attacks the wrong thing, or fails to attack anything at all. Scientists have been looking at the reasons for this, and many now believe that there may be more to the story than bad lifestyle choices. The answer, or at least part of it, may lie in the dramatic depletion of what is now known as the microbiome.

A large proportion of the cells in the human body are not human cells at all, but microbial organisms – bacteria, viruses, fungi and protozoa. They support and interact with the human cells to allow the natural processes and functions of our bodies to take place and this collection of essential organisms is called the microbiome. All life on earth has evolved from and with bacteria, and a complex ecosystem exists both inside and outside our bodies. We provide a habitat for bacteria, and in return they regulate our metabolism and play an essential role in setting up our immune system.

There are around 400 species of bacteria found in the vagina alone. As a baby passes through the birth canal, he receives a dose of his mother's bacteria along the way. If he is then placed on her body in skin-to-skin contact he receives further microbial colonisation. The third stage in the process is the initiation of breastfeeding, which is stimulated by neonatal reflexes in response to skin contact (we'll get to that in the next chapter). Breastmilk contains antibodies and anti-inflammatories that help to set up the baby's immune system, as well as oligosaccharides (sugars), which also play a crucial role.

Until recently, the presence of these particular sugars in breastmilk was a mystery, because the baby cannot digest them. It was only when the importance of 'good' bacteria for gut function started to become apparent, that the purpose of the oligosaccharides became clear. For example, the bacteria *Lactobacillus bifidus* makes the gut more acidic, thus helping to stop 'bad' bacteria from growing. The oligosaccharides feed the newly seeded good bacterial colonies, ensuring their survival. This is one of the reasons why extended breastfeeding contributes to the development of a strong immune system. 'The initial colonisation of the intestine is a moment of pivotal importance in long-term health, playing a profound role in imprinting of immune and systematic homeostasis.'[49]

The development of a symbiotic relationship between specific bacteria and the baby's immune system has gradually evolved over millions of years, and it is only in the last century that we have routinely removed some or all of the crucial stages in the process that sets it up (vaginal birth, skin-to-skin contact and breastfeeding). It is now hypothesised that in doing so, we have unwittingly altered the balance of our internal microbiomes, and the consequences of this are yet to become clear. It is estimated that through the use of antibiotics we have already lost approximately a third of the human microbiome, and that just like removing a third of the trees from a forest, the whole ecosystem is put under stress by the loss of diversity. Ultimately, there is the potential for it to collapse.

The bacteria a baby is exposed to during vaginal birth are almost always harmless. They form the basis of the baby's immune system because they will 'teach' it which bacteria should be tolerated and which should be attacked. Seeding the baby with good bacteria is essential for creating the internal balance of microbes that is needed for good health, and the window of opportunity for this to occur is remarkably brief. It needs to happen early on in the baby's development if the immune system is to fully mature. Later exposure to good bacteria may go some way to make up for the loss, but in many individuals, the immune system will simply have the wrong programming and may never be fully able to distinguish between good and bad cells.

The significance of this may be enormous. Our interference with our microbiome could potentially have implications for the future health of the entire human race, because by reducing our internal bacterial diversity we are potentially weakening our immune systems. Caesareans are believed to have played a large part in this story because they frequently cause an interruption to the natural post-partum period, making breastfeeding more problematic. Not only does this have an impact on initial bacterial colonisation, but it also makes antibiotic use more likely in future, because formula-fed babies are at higher risk of infections. So while we are encouraging more virulent and antibiotic-resistant strains of bad bacteria to evolve, through the misuse and overuse of antibiotics, we are also weakening our ability to fight them by failing to correctly seed our microbiomes.

In situations where a caesarean is unavoidable, it has been suggested that a vaginal swab should be taken from the mother, which could be applied to the baby immediately after delivery.

This, combined with immediate skin-to-skin contact and full-term breastfeeding, would ensure the correct development of his immune system. These are important factors for healthcare providers to consider when deciding what the future of maternity care should be.[50]

Whether birth takes place on an operating table, in the bath or on the bus, it is invariably a crossroads in life, at which we can find ourselves to be empowered or disempowered. Birth is an everyday event, a normal human bodily function, but your experience of it will cast long shadows into the future of your family, so it does matter. Birth is a private conversation between a mother and baby, but everyone who loves them depends on the success of this exchange and the burgeoning relationship that follows. Romeo said of Juliet, 'nothing can be ill if she be well'[51] and indeed, nothing can be well, if she be ill. A mother traumatised by childbirth carries a heavy burden which threatens the happiness of her whole family. Everyone involved in the birth, be they midwife, doctor, father, doula or grandmother, has a responsibility to play a *supporting* role to the mother. Her needs and wishes matter more than anyone or anything else in the room. Within that microcosm, the mother is the sun and everything revolves around her. So laminate your birth plan. Assert yourself. And if you cannot, then enlist someone else to be your advocate. Your experience of birth matters now and for the rest of your life.

4. MILK

If you look into your own heart, and you find nothing wrong there, what is there to worry about? What is there to fear?
– Confucius

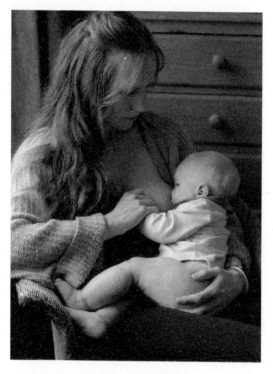

I) THE GOLDEN HOUR

When a woman reaches out and gathers her newborn baby into her arms, she will almost always bring him to her chest and lie back to rest. Believe it or not, this is as far as a mother's instincts go when it comes to breastfeeding, and to some extent, it is actually all that is required at the start. From there, the reflexes and instincts that initiate human breastfeeding behaviour come from the baby. It may seem incredible, but research is now uncovering an obvious truth that may go some way to explain why so many women don't find breastfeeding comes naturally to them. Breastfeeding on the part of the mother is a learnt art that is handed down from one generation to the next and relies on the ability to see it in action from an early age. But a baby comes with the necessary reflexes and instincts built in, because he doesn't have the option of learning what to do. And these instincts kick in immediately after birth. You could say that birth and breastfeeding are part of the same process.

It can be deeply upsetting to find that breastfeeding does not come naturally and I know from experience the crippling feelings of shame and disappointment that take hold when it turns out to be a struggle. It is easy to feel that we are no good if we don't instinctively know what to do, but that is far from the truth. It may be that we are looking at things from the wrong perspective and expecting too much of ourselves. We have come to believe that it is our job to initiate breastfeeding, because we believe that babies are helpless, but that is not entirely true. Painkillers that pass through the placenta during labour and make our babies sleepy, as well as a multitude of post-birth interventions often rob them of the opportunity to show us what they can do. The Golden Hour after birth is a pivotal moment and separating mothers and babies at this point, even for a short time, inadvertently interrupts an important natural process, and can throw a great big spanner in the works for successful breastfeeding.

In the 1950s and 60s more and more women were starting to have their babies in hospitals rather than at home, and separation immediately after birth became commonplace. Babies were weighed, checked, cleaned and their eyes were treated with silver nitrate drops before being taken to the nursery as an 'infection control' precaution. Bottle-feeding was routine in these nurseries and formula milk came as part of the package that was 'modern' baby care. Babies survived birth and got fed, everyone breathed a sigh of relief, and no one noticed that anything was amiss. Although hospitals in the UK no longer despatch newborn babies to a nursery, it is still standard practice for disruptive procedures to be carried out soon after birth. A baby's first hour on earth often involves being handed from one person to the next, and very little stillness or intimacy in connection with his mother. But the idea that this might cause problems with bonding and breastfeeding has only recently begun to hold weight.

It appears that breastfeeding has always been considered something that happens some time after birth. But to get off to a good start, we really need to think of it as a part of birth – a crucial link in a chain of events that does not stop once the baby is born. Just as we now recognise that a fourth trimester takes place outside the womb, due to the big head/small pelvis issue we discussed earlier, so too is there is a fourth stage to birth. It is the immediate reinstatement of the physical bond between mother and baby and it marks the beginning of the fourth trimester. Breastfeeding is a continuation of the symbiosis that exists between mother and baby during pregnancy. This relationship will evolve over the course of the months and years that follow as the child's physical need for his mother diminishes, but whoever severs the bond that connects them during pregnancy by catching the baby and cutting the cord is responsible for reconnecting them straight away and initiating this relationship. A mother still nourishes and protects her baby with her body.

When placed on his mother's abdomen straight after birth, a baby will often take to her breast and begin to suckle before the placenta has been expelled. Suckling stimulates prolactin to release the placenta and tie off blood vessels to prevent haemorrhage, so it is clearly an important part of nature's plan for birth. If the cord is not cut immediately, then the bond can be reformed before it has even been broken. When birth attendants recognise the importance of this transition and allow mothers and babies to be together, undisturbed for at least the first hour after birth, the chances of a positive outcome for women who would like to breastfeed can be radically improved.

But most of us have little or no idea what this scene should look like, or what we should be doing. Two years after the birth of my first baby, I was sitting in a children's centre surrounded by other trainee breastfeeding peer supporters, watching a documentary film. It was just a few minutes long, but I could hardly believe what played out on the screen in front of me. A naked, newborn baby was placed on his mother's bare abdomen and simply left there. For a few minutes he wriggled around as you might expect, but it soon became clear that his movements were not random. The baby was pushing his feet against his mother's thighs and moving towards her breasts. Once his nose reached one breast he began bobbing his head until he found the nipple and, having found his 'target' (this is why our nipples become darker during pregnancy), he stopped for a short rest before beginning again. He opened wide, latched on deeply and began to suckle. He had done it by himself. You couldn't ask for better positioning and attachment. My jaw was on the floor.

Babies are born with reflexes. Around 10 of these have been identified and some emerge later on during development, so it is thought that they may serve different functions at different times. But the purpose of these reflexes is not always obvious and it is sometimes thought that they played a role in our ancestral past but are no longer useful. Many paediatricians have puzzled over the newborn stepping reflex which is present at birth but soon disappears. Babies are not able to hold their own weight at birth, and are by no means ready to walk, so what could it be for? Is it possible that, when combined with a couple of other reflexes, it contributes to the initiation of breastfeeding? The stepping reflex helps the baby to push forwards and find the breast, the rooting reflex helps him find the nipple and the sucking reflex allows him to begin nursing. You have to admit it makes sense.

We are not surprised to see a newborn animal instinctively seek out his food source, but it goes against the way we think about 'helpless' human babies for them to do this too. It's called the 'breast crawl', and if a baby is not drowsy from a medicated or traumatic birth, he will almost always make an attempt at it. But the window of opportunity is short. If it does not happen within the first hour, it is unlikely to happen at all. Unfortunately many mothers will attempt their first feed only after the rigmarole of post-birth procedures is over. When everyone has been tidied up, stitched up and bundled up, we hold our babies tentatively and offer them the breast. Not entirely sure what to do or how to do it, we often end up with a poor latch that needs work.

Dr Christina Smillie is a paediatrician and board-certified lactation consultant whose research has led her to describe breastfeeding as a right-brain activity, like riding a bicycle. If you were suddenly presented with a bike and had never seen anyone riding one before, what are the chances you would know what to do? We need to watch someone else before trying it ourselves and then we need to practise at it in order to learn. The trouble is there are so few opportunities to get a good look at breastfeeding or even to talk about it these days. Most of the time we are playing it blind.[1]

Ina May Gaskin has observed successful initiation of breastfeeding thousands of times, but even in the early days of her practice, before the Golden Hour had been given a name, the implications of insensitive obstetrical care were obvious to her. In *Spiritual Midwifery*, she writes:

'The period of time directly following birth is a time of extremely heightened sensitivity for both the mother and her infant. Deep psychic grooves are being cut in the consciousness of both which will drastically affect later behaviour, especially in the mother's ability to care for her young [...] Research has shown that interference with the normal bonding process has a great and sometimes drastic impact on the family. This exactly corroborates our own observations [...] Klaus and Kennell's [1976] studies showed that women who had their babies with them immediately after birth, who were allowed skin-to-skin contact, undisturbed for a while, held their babies more competently, established more intimate contact with their babies, and had fewer problems with breastfeeding than mothers who were separated from their babies immediately following birth and rejoined later. It seems that this mothering ability is greatly affected by how freely the mother is able to follow her own instinctual sense.'[2]

But all is not lost. There is a style of breastfeeding that echoes the breast crawl and encourages the baby's natural feeding reflexes and helps promote a good latch. It's called biological nurturing and Suzanne Colson is a midwife with a PhD for her research into this style of 'laid-back breastfeeding'. She says:

'Human neonates are born with an innate ability to find the breast, latch and feed. Unfortunately, some of these very reflexes can also hinder babies' efforts to breastfeed depending on the mother's posture [...] our findings suggest that when mothers sit upright, or even when they lie on their sides, gravity pulls the baby away from the mother's body [potentially causing muscle strain and nipple damage for the mother and poor milk transfer for the baby [...] As soon as mothers lie back, they look comfortable, relaxed and focused upon their babies – often smiling, giggling and oblivious to the world. The baby finds the breast using his inborn reflexes that now look smooth and purposeful. Because the strength of reaction is somewhat blunted by gravity, the baby reflexes appear to aid neonatal locomotion leading to latching behaviours, self attachment and good milk transfer.'[3]

Nursing a baby in the upright feeding position we are usually taught often causes us to lean forwards and strain our backs.

The weight of the baby is hard to manage for long periods and our arms are not free to do anything else. Newborns feed often and for long periods of time, drifting in and out of sleep, so the inconvenience and discomfort we may experience makes this hard to endure and hard to believe that this it is how it is supposed to be. It feels all wrong, but we are told we must learn to manage the feeds better and then put the baby down. Laid-back breastfeeding in the early days after birth allows the mother and baby to relax without the pressure of perfecting the hold straight away. We can rest comfortably and the baby can feed and sleep most of the time. It doesn't mean we can't get up and do other things if we need to, but while we are together, we are in a happy place.

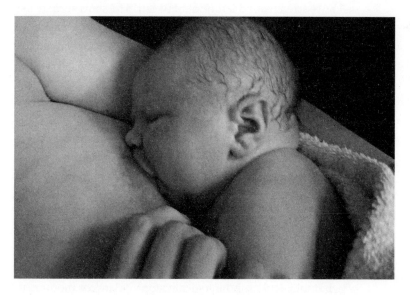

Biological nurturing is also helpful for mothers with a forceful let-down reflex. Many babies choke, 'click' and splutter at the start of a feed, when the milk is flowing fast and this can cause problems like reflux and trapped wind. But when the mother reclines, gravity holds the milk back a little and the baby can often manage things better. (This does not inhibit a normal let-down reflex; it will still allow for efficient milk transfer when the flow is not fast.) Many babies also love lying on their tummy, in full-body contact. It is a delicious way to take a nap, but like so many of the nice things to do with babies, we are often told that this is a bad habit and not to be encouraged. Well, it's time to bury that old chestnut. Arm yourself with the knowledge that biological nurturing is so called because it is exactly how babies have nursed and slept throughout the course of our evolutionary history, and they still do it in many cultures today. This position is safe, comfortable, minimises reflux and promotes baby-led feeding patterns.

Being comfortable is vitally important for breastfeeding on cue because if you are dreading the next feed, the temptation will be to stretch out the time in between. The short-term result of this is a ravenous baby who might pull hard on engorged breasts, or struggle to latch on. But in the long term, stretching out feeds can cause the milk ducts to become blocked, leading to mastitis and ultimately a reduction in milk production. Producing the right amount of milk for your baby relies on a feedback system of supply and demand which primes the breasts to produce the right amount. Production can go up as well as down. The more often the brain receives the message that the baby is feeding the more milk will be produced. It is the frequency rather than the duration of feeds that provides this feedback and this counts at night just as much as during the day, so we should be thinking of nursing as a 24-hour commitment.

Although generally low in fat, human milk has been shown to have a higher fat content when feeding intervals are kept short, which implies that it is biologically appropriate for mothers to sleep close to their babies and feed them throughout the night. It is the fat in breastmilk that is the key ingredient for brain development, and a lot of that brain work goes on at night, when the day's events are being processed and new pathways are being laid down. In the light of this, the idea that babies can 'go without' the calories for 12 hours becomes irrelevant. Babies are not just body-building at night, they are brain-building, and they need fuel to do it. Anthropologist Meredith Small describes the natural human feeding style as follows:

> 'When the milk is low in fat and protein as it is in humans, it is an indication that breast-feeding is designated or intended to be more continuous. Human milk is 88 percent water and 4.5 percent fat on average, depending on the style of feeding; interval feeding with long spaces in between produces lower-fat milk, while continuous feeding produces higher-fat milk.'[4]

So having the right proportion of fat in the milk is important not only because it is satisfying for the baby and less likely to cause intestinal discomfort, but because it is the long-chain fatty acids in breastmilk that myelinate (insulate) the baby's newly developing nerve cells. Frequent feeding also ensures a higher overall fat content in the milk, because fat is re-absorbed from the milk back into the mother's body in between feeds while it sits in the breasts. As a feed progresses, fat globules are slowly released back into the milk.[5] This accounts for the sweet, watery foremilk present at the beginning of a feed. The longer the gap between feeds the more foremilk there will be. Fat is added in as the feed goes on, so for the milk to contain the right balance, we need to feed our babies frequently.

It is depressingly common for women to think that they are not producing enough milk, or that their milk is not of good quality. But the recommendations to feed babies every two–three hours and for a limited time (along with warnings like, 'don't let your baby use you as a dummy') essentially ensure this very outcome. A top-up of formula is usually the next 'logical' step, and a snowball effect, sometimes resulting in 'failure' to breastfeed is often quick to follow. But this is in our heads as much as it is in our bodies, and it is impossible to underestimate the power of cultural influence. A consultant midwife once told me about a woman she'd cared for who had had three children: 'The first two were born and breastfed in Bangladesh but she had her third child in the UK and was mix-feeding. When asked why she was giving her baby formula she replied that she believed she did not have enough milk, although she laughed when she realised what she'd said.'[6] The fact that upon arrival in the UK this woman had started to doubt her body's ability to make milk speaks volumes about the way that our cultural message undermines women's belief in their bodies.

Meredith Small points out that around the world 'breasts come in all sorts of shapes and sizes, and it seems that there is no relationship between shape or size and what the breast can do'.[7] Insufficient glandular tissue, damage from surgery or hormonal imbalances relating to polycystic ovaries or thyroid abnormalities can cause major problems with milk production. But according to a recent study, even the amount of glandular (milk-making) tissue in the breasts, which is often called into question when women struggle with breastfeeding, could be irrelevant unless it is missing altogether. The study used ultrasound imaging to look at the amount of glandular tissue in breasts of all different shapes and sizes, and concluded that 'breast morphology was not predictive of the internal anatomy of the breast'.[8] You can't externally assess how much glandular tissue a woman has, and breast size is not related to milk production or storage ability because large breasts are for storing fat, not milk. Not only that, having less glandular tissue does not necessarily mean that you produce less milk, it simply means that the baby will feed more frequently to extract the same amount. It is only in a culture that frowns on frequent feeding where this becomes a problem.

Apart from cases of outright famine, it appears that different ethnic groups also manage to feed their babies perfectly adequately, even when nutrition is less than ideal. If necessary, the mother's body will always draw on stores within itself, to manufacture the ingredients for making milk. A study on mothers in Gambia, West Africa revealed that contrary to the researchers' expectations, supplementing the diet of a group of mothers did *not* increase the volume or quality of the milk they produced. The only effect was that some of them started ovulating again. The body will always look after the existing baby, and additional nutrition just makes it possible for the mother to have another one.[9]

In many places where breastfeeding is considered the normal way to feed a baby, the idea of feeding 'on demand' would not even be understood. If anything, it might be described as feeding 'on cue', but mothers who do not feel compelled to monitor how or when their babies feed are likely to have a completely different way of thinking about it.

'Infants are not demanding anything and mothers are not giving in; the baby is simply feeding. Infants of hunter-gatherers feed very frequently. Botswanan !Kung San infants, for example, feed every thirteen minutes on average. This pattern of frequent feeding, with the infant soon able to guide the process himself, probably echoes how the first human infants fed until they were able to walk, some time during the first year or so. Human infants long ago must have also been carried all the time; they probably slept with their mothers and fed frequently throughout the day and night. In fact during 99 per cent of human history this was surely the pattern of infant eating, sleeping and contact. The current pattern in some cultures of long intervals between feeding, no night feeding, and supplementation of mother's milk with other species' milk or artificial milk is very recent for the human species.'[10]

The idea of feeding a baby every 13 minutes may sound absurd or impossible, and I'm not suggesting that this is something we should all be doing. But it might help to assuage any worries about feeding babies 'too often'. In comparison to this, feeding every 90 minutes almost sounds ungenerous! The !Kung San women feed their babies and do not give a thought to when, why or how much. So the old argument that 'he can't be hungry again', whether true or not, is irrelevant. 'The German word for breastfeeding, *stillen*, means to quieten and soothe rather than to give food.'[11] In English, 'nursing' conveys an element of comforting, which is why I actually prefer this to the word 'breastfeeding'. It's not just a mechanical means of survival but an emotionally enriching one as well. Breastmilk is digested very rapidly and frequent feeds provide a bundle of benefits: the baby's blood sugar remains level, the milk stays rich and satisfying, the mother's breasts remain soft and comfortable and a moment of comfort in the big bad world is never far away. There are a whole host of reasons why frequent feeding is appropriate for babies, but new mothers who may lack knowledge or confidence in this are vulnerable to those haunting words 'don't let him use you as a dummy'.

II) WHO ARE YOU CALLING DUMMY?

They say it takes a village to raise a child. In non-industrialised cultures, where breastfeeding is practised in a more or less continuous fashion, babies are usually born into a large family group within a close community. The mother would never be left alone with a baby for ten hours of the day, and there are plenty of willing hands, ready to share the task and take the baby for a while. A mother can enjoy short breaks in between feeds and this balances the needs of the baby with her own. Western mothers, on the other hand, are often the sole provider of physical contact throughout the day for our babies and it is a heavy burden to bear. Many women will identify with the feeling of wanting to hand the baby over the minute their partner steps through the door. And the thought of even more physical contact at the end of a long day is often too much to bear, so many relationships take a hard knock. Fathers can often feel rejected and resentful.

As Mei-Ling Hopgood points out in *How Eskimos Keep Their Babies Warm*, the modern nuclear family falls short of our evolutionary social requirements: '[W]e evolved as cooperative breeders. To survive, human babies needed not only their mothers but also a tribe of support that included the father, and grandparents, siblings, aunts, and other relatives and friends.'[12] She goes on to describe how the fathers in the Aka pygmy tribes of Central Africa offer mothers considerable relief from a baby's physical needs. From the start, they will offer their own nipples to suck and the babies accept this as an alternative to the mother, even though there is no milk. The Aka are a very peaceful people, and since the men have no call to go to war, a strong bond between fathers and their children is encouraged. The men will happily sit together, chatting and working, while suckling and cuddling their babies. If they have to go anywhere, the father is more likely to carry the child than the mother because he is physically stronger. The gender roles are distinguishable, but the tasks assigned to them are interchangeable.[13]

Many parents in industrialised nations adopt a different means to the same end. We offer our babies a dummy (or pacifier). Sometimes this works well and makes life easier for busy mothers who want their babies to settle on their own. But many babies refuse a dummy and many mothers feel uncomfortable about using them. I have been told on more than one occasion that by allowing my baby to comfort feed I am being used as a human pacifier. But a dummy is a substitute for a human, not the other way around. My babies were happy to suck my baby finger, but they had no interest in a dummy. Just remember that when it comes to 'essential' baby products like dummies, there is someone out there making money from perpetuating the idea that our bodies aren't enough.

A dummy is just another piece in the puzzle that when you put it all together spells out 'put the baby down'. If that is what the baby wants then fine, but if not, then I would always argue that comfort in the form of human contact is superior to anything else. As the example of the Aka pygmy men shows, parents and carers who do not make milk can still be an essential source of comfort to their babies and we could do to adjust our preconceptions. The SNS (supplemental nursing system) is an amazing piece of equipment which takes this idea a step further by allowing a baby to draw milk from a bottle through a flexible straw that can be taped to the nipple. Unlike many other artificial feeding products, this one actually promotes attachment and reinforces the important role of the parent or carer in every different feeding scenario.

The fact that we are willing and able to address our babies' needs with our bodies is something to be proud of, not ashamed of. But somehow we are made to question this, and to question whether comfort can even be put into the same category of 'need' as food. We try to divide the two, but this makes no sense in the real world. If a child falls over we wouldn't put a plaster on and refuse to give him a hug. Physical and emotional needs at times of distress are of equal importance. Babies need comfort to feel alive and well, just as much as they need food to stay alive and well. We are not creating 'comfort eaters' when we offer the breast. We are merely providing reassurance that everything is in order and all is well.

III) LIQUID GOLD

Colostrum, or 'liquid gold', as it is sometimes called, is the first milk that the breasts produce immediately after birth (although some women notice it starts to emerge from their nipples in the late stages of pregnancy). High in protein, protective lysozymes and immunoglobulin, it is the ideal food for a newborn baby. It provides an immediate inoculation against harmful pathogens and is a highly concentrated energy source for the first few days. It is a natural laxative and allows the baby to pass their thick, dark meconium stools quickly, and clear out their gut. A full-term newborn baby is born with extra fluid on board, which is enough to see him through the first few days. And his stomach starts out the size of a cherry, so tiny amounts of concentrated food are all that he requires.

Nature has evolved a perfect solution for the specific needs of the newborn. There is nothing that can be done to improve on what has been provided. But compared with the image of a full bottle of pure white milk, many mothers can't help questioning the value of these little droplets of yellow liquid. In many cultures around the world it is customary for mothers to be told to wait for the 'proper' milk to come in, before commencing breastfeeding. As a result, the first thing that happens to millions of babies upon entry into the world is the deprivation of one of the most nutritionally important meals of their entire lives. No other animal on the planet chooses to do this. When it comes to breastfeeding, we think too much.

IV) THE MAGIC FORMULA

Let me start by saying that I am not pro- or anti-breastfeeding. I am not pro- or anti-formula-feeding. I am in favour of all babies being nourished and cared for so that both mother and baby can thrive. In a country with poor levels of sanitation and resources, the safest and healthiest option is almost invariably to breastfeed. In Western societies, where exclusive, full-term breastfeeding is no longer understood or considered normal, a baby may need to be formula-fed in order to do well. For some mothers it comes as a great relief to end their struggles with breastfeeding and to give their baby a bottle. For others, it is important to have an alternative available to them from day one. Their right to bottle-feed is as important as any other right relating to women's bodies, and it is a choice we should be able to make without judgement. But our choices are influenced by our cultural environment, so a problem arises when these choices are not fairly informed. And, unfortunately, it is often very hard to distinguish information from advertising.

Even if you have no doubt in your mind about how you

intend to feed your baby, I am willing to bet that it turns out to be more complicated than you expect. I struggled with breastfeeding first time around and I know how hard it can be. My attempts with bottles were equally fraught and ended in failure (a faulty steriliser, an aversion to 'pumping' and an unfortunate bottle-melted-in-saucepan-incident put an end to all of that). Feeding babies is a skill that must be learnt, and most mothers have to learn on the job. It is not just about calories going in. It involves countless decisions about how, what and when you feed the baby. Today these decisions are influenced by market forces and societal pressures. Very few of us ever make truly informed choices when it comes to feeding our children, because our collective common knowledge has so many gaping holes in it. Food manufacturers have replaced inherited wisdom and common sense, with misinformation, fearmongering and manipulative marketing propaganda. Nestlé describes itself as 'the world's leading health, wellness and nutrition company' and in the same paragraph lists some of its most popular products: Kit Kat, Nescafé, Smarties and Shreddies.[14] These are not health foods by any stretch of the imagination. The simple truths about good food are largely hidden from view, because they are not financially profitable. And food industry marketing has infiltrated our healthcare system to such an extent that it is woven into the advice we are given by professionals. We are bombarded by mixed messages and can be left feeling guilty, powerless and bewildered.

We are told that 'Breast is Best' but the sad truth is that when breastfeeding is not properly supported or correctly practised, as is often the case in technologically advanced societies, it can actually be detrimental to the physical and mental well-being of mothers and babies. Our ability to provide what our babies need is routinely questioned and our confidence is undermined. Our bodies may be deemed capable enough while our babies are still inside us, but once they emerge into the outside world, our ability to continue to nurture them is immediately and inexplicably called into question. Once formula has been given to a baby, often on the advice of healthcare professionals, it can be extremely difficult to go back to exclusive breastfeeding and concerns about 'insufficient milk supply' become self-fulfilling. Mothers who wish to breastfeed but who were not well supported or informed from the outset should never be made to feel that they have failed to do the best for their babies. In these instances, it is healthcare providers and society as a whole that are failing everyone.

Let's face it, when it comes to parenting we are *all* searching for the perfect formula. We are all looking for the magic ingredients – we want to 'get it right'. The name of the product that exploits this need most fiercely is no coincidence. The very word 'formula' is a shrewd play on our deepest desires. It conjures ideas of scientific precision, of correctness and perfection. But it's an illusion. Manufactured milk is in no way better, or anywhere near as complete for human babies as human milk. While human milk has perfected itself over thousands of years of evolution, formula is a relatively recent experiment into infant nutrition and it has miraculously carved a niche for itself where one previously did not exist. The ubiquity of this product both implies and answers the 'need' for itself. Would we need formula so much if it weren't so readily available?

Artificial milk may have been needed to feed orphans and strays, but formula as we know it today was developed as a commercial product and from the very beginning it was marketed to all infants, not just to those who really needed it. In 1865, chemist Justus von Liebig developed, patented and marketed the first genuinely effective human milk substitute. Von Liebig's formula (consisting of cow's milk, wheat flour, malt flour, pea flour and bicarbonate of potash), was promoted as the perfect infant food.[15] But von Liebig was annoyed when doctors reported that his food was indigestible and questioned whether it was as good as human milk. He wrote, 'If we were to say that this preparation does not agree with new-born babies, such a statement could not be supported on theoretical grounds, since in the food they get the very same ingredients as mother's milk.'[16] He may have been deluded, but he was certainly determined and was not to be deterred.

It seems unlikely that you could sell a product so successfully if there was no need for it, but formula marketing taps into a deep well of emotional insecurity. Everyone wants what is best for their children, and women are at their most vulnerable when they are becoming new mothers. It is hard to accept that something as seemingly benign and innocent as baby milk has the potential to be damaging in any way, but the murky world of human milk substitution is a disturbing one, and it is shocking to discover there are other motivations for the promotion of formula milk than a baby's health and well-being.

They all claim to be the 'best', but many of the formula brands that appear to be different from one another, such as Aptamil and Cow & Gate, are made in the same factories and from the same ingredients. Indeed, the ingredients of formula milk are so tightly regulated that there is scarcely any difference at all between them. There is also no significant compositional difference between infant milk and so-called 'follow-on' or 'growing-up' milk. In fact, it is worth noting that this 'second-stage' milk only emerged within the industry as a result of changing legislation that laid out strict new advertising parameters (Infant Formula and Follow-on Formula (England) Regulations 2007). In an effort to promote breastfeeding, the legislation prohibits any claims that babies 'need' formula. But it seems that, far from deterring the formula companies, these changes spurred them on to produce more creative branding and ad campaigns. Advertisements adopted slogans, such as 'Do I look like I'm not getting everything I need?', that subtly promote the idea that formula competes with breastmilk on equal grounds. Aptamil taps into the aspirational hopes of parents using scientific, futuristic branding and its ads depict babies' future selves as astronauts, athletes and ballerinas. It sells an even greater promise than a satisfied baby. It sells success.

These companies also prey on the insecurities of parents who fear that their babies aren't getting 'enough', whether because they are bigger than average or smaller than average. We are often told that babies sleep for longer when they are 'properly' satisfied and we believe that long sleeps are 'best'. We can be easily convinced that there is a problem. The branding of 'hungry-baby' milk implies that it is more nourishing than regular milk (be it formula or breastmilk), but hungry-baby milk actually contains no extra calories. Instead it contains a slightly higher proportion of protein, which means it takes longer to digest and babies who drink it will appear to be full for longer. This is a problem not only because babies may take in less energy overall if they are fed less often, but the type of energy their bodies get will be incorrect because human milk is naturally low in protein. A major study recently identified a link between childhood obesity and excessive protein intake during the first two years of a child's life.[17] The trouble is that newborn babies need more protein than older babies and while the protein levels in breastmilk change organically over time, reducing by about a third by week four, protein levels in formula are relatively high to ensure they meet the needs of a newborn baby. By 10 to 12 weeks postpartum, breastmilk contains half as much protein as it did during the newborn stage; but in spite of offering a range of milks for different 'stages', all formula generally tends to have a higher protein content than breastmilk overall.

V) PAYING THE PRICE:
A LAND OF MILK AND HONEYS

The commodification of women is nothing new. Women's bodies have been 'owned' throughout history. But in today's world of pop stars, porn stars and Page Three girls, a woman's breasts have been reassigned from the functional yet beautiful asset that they once were to a purely aesthetic kind of trophy.

Women have been 'liberated' from the burden of breastfeeding, but our breasts are linked with our worth as much as they ever have been, if not more than ever before. And this value can be transferred to any given product through a woman's association with it. It's a marketing strategy that sells cars, newspapers, movies and a cultural ideal of youth and perfection that has us frowning in the mirror and reaching for our credit cards. In the world of commodity, there is always something new and improved on the market and by rendering our breasts obsolete we have made them as dispensable as any other product. We can buy better breasts from a surgeon or bra manufacturer; and we can buy milk to feed our babies on every high street in the country.

We have literally been conditioned by our consumerist culture to judge our own milk by the packaging it comes in. We are led to believe that what our bodies produce has the same, if not less, value than what we see packaged on the shelves. The formula industry plays on the underlying acceptance that women's bodies are inadequate, dispensable and intrinsically connected to commerce but most of us do not even realise the way that formula marketing plays on our insecurities and undermines our self-worth. 'Failure to breastfeed', as it is commonly described, is not a failure at all but an injustice. It is a common problem that arises above all from misinformation and environmental conditioning. Women are robbed of the right to fulfil their body's potential before they are even aware of wanting to do so. We are programmed by society to believe that we are inadequate and by the time we come to use our breasts for the purpose for which they exist, we have already learnt to judge them according to a standard which is based on form over function. We are surrounded by messages of perfection, and all too often the conclusion we come to is that we do not measure up.

Having been primed to think that our bodies are no good, we are more susceptible to the formula industry's message that the milk we produce is not necessary anyway. Why bother when the products on the shelves guarantee a healthy baby? It's hard to picture a male-orientated equivalent to the cultural wallpaper of augmented, unrealistic breasts that women are subjected to, but let's try for a minute. Imagine a world where men were surrounded by images of swollen penises bulging between muscular thighs. Not just tucked neatly into underwear, but on show and impossible to avoid. What if, when the time came for a man to make a child, he was told that if he couldn't manage to ejaculate, there was a product available in the shops that could do the job just as well? Not an expensive product, but a mass-produced and affordable one that worked every time and guaranteed a healthy baby. It changes things a bit. How might that make him feel? Uncomfortable? A little doubt might creep in. Would he take pride in his role or might he feel that it was somehow self-indulgent to carry out his purpose. Of course nobody would ever consider that product equal to the real thing. But make no mistake, we cannot replicate human milk any more than we can replicate semen. It is unique to our species, and it is alive.

Human milk contains around a hundred constituents that cannot be replicated or preserved in formula milk, with more being discovered all the time.[18] They include stem cells that have the potential to become any kind of cell the body needs for growth and repair; lymphocytes, T-cells, leukocytes, lysozyme, cytokines, mucin, lactoferrin and immunoglobulin, which all play key roles in the immune system; alpha-lactalbumin and linoleic acid, which have anti-cancer properties; growth factors; nucleotides; hormones and anti-inflammatory components. Most recently, scientists have found that lactoferrin may hold the key to fighting antibiotic-resistant superbugs.[19] The discovery of all these properties has meant that breastmilk is now valuable for medical research. Human milk sells on the Internet for about £2 per ounce (roughly 260 times the price of oil); for such an abundant commodity, it has an astonishingly high value. But this value is only realised under certain circumstances and to certain people, because a woman breastfeeding her own children has never counted towards the economy in any measurable or acknowledgeable way. The formula companies would have us believe that it is pointless, worthless and unnecessary.

The list of living elements in human milk is pretty incredible and one of the most recent discoveries is its anti-cancer properties:

'Researchers have recently identified a tiny peptide called lactaptin derived from breast milk that destroys cancer cells and leaves healthy ones alive. [And] in 2010, researchers found that the substance in breast milk known as Hamlet (Human Alpha-lactalbumin Made LEthal to Tumour) cells could be used to kill 40 different types of cancer. Hamlet is produced by combining alpha-lactalbumin in the milk and oleic acid which is found in babies' stomachs. So breast milk could well be preventive of cancer in babies.'[20]

Everything to do with human milk has been culturally pasteurised. The language we use to describe breastfeeding has become so prosaic that all trace of the human, emotional or even spiritual aspects of nourishing our babies has been steam-cleaned out of our vocabulary. It's fine to talk about health benefits, saving money and saving the planet, but we tend to be matter-of-fact about things like 'bonding', in case it invokes discomfort, ridicule or condemnation. Our uncertainty about the value of our milk is compounded by its commodification and we end up talking about our bodies as though we were a production line. We talk about our 'supply', as though our milk were in need of constant monitoring lest it run out. Another job for mothers to add to an already long and tedious list. It's all fine as long as we get on with it discreetly and don't make too much of a scene.

Milk does work on a supply-and-demand basis, but we need not fret about stock check or logistics. Given half a chance our bodies and our babies can work this out between themselves. But it seems that suspicion arises whenever anything cannot be precisely quantified or controlled. Patriarchy will not allow for women to have control of something significant, powerful and unquantifiable. Our milk is being put under the microscope, analysed and its secrets are being unlocked. The magic in the milk is being unravelled, stripped down and catalogued into its component pieces before being reformulated and fed back into our culture in sterile blister packs. We are using breastmilk to create drugs that do the job of breastmilk. The difference is that someone can make money from it if it comes in a pill.

Breastmilk is protective against many diseases including leukaemia, type 1 diabetes, ear and respiratory infections, diarrhoea, meningitis, sudden unexplained death in infants (SUDI) and necrotising enterocolitis.[21] Mounting evidence suggests that conditions such as inflammatory bowel syndrome, juvenile diabetes, breast cancer and malignant lymphoma are linked to being bottle-fed as an infant. Chronic conditions, such as asthma, allergies and middle ear infections, are certainly more common in children and adults who were bottle-fed.[22] But in spite of all of this, most babies in developed countries who are formula-fed appear to do just fine, largely because we have the resources to use formula safely and to deal with any health problems that it may create. But formula companies do not limit their sights to mothers in affluent countries. In fact, their marketing strategies are often more aggressive in poorer countries, where regulations may be less stringent or harder to enforce.

Mothers in developing nations are extremely vulnerable to manipulation. Like everyone else, they want the best for their children. If they see or are told that babies in affluent societies are often fed formula, they will believe that they should try to do the same. The cost of formula itself is crippling and formula is often over-diluted to make it stretch further; but once a mother's milk has dried up there is no alternative, so the milk must be paid for and older children may have to go hungry. Using unpotable water to make it up is also very common in poor countries. When fuel is a major drain on a household's resources, it is impossible to light the fire for five sterile feeds a day; and in areas with unsafe water, a bottle-fed child is up to 25 times more likely to die as a result of diarrhoea.[23] But formula manufacturer Nestlé won't stop at selling milk. In many parts of the world, they are working towards controlling water supplies so that people might soon have to pay for the clean water they need to make up the formula as well. In 2013, Nestlé CEO Peter Brabeck stated, 'NGOs bang on about declaring water is a public right. That means that as a human being you should have a right to water. That's an extreme answer [...] water is a foodstuff like any other, and like any other foodstuff it should have a market value.'[24] It's much easier to say this when you are rich than when you have no money for food, let alone water.

We may sometimes feel that the troubles of poor people in far-off lands are not really our fault or concern. But we humans are all connected on many levels, across continents, whether we see it or not. The richest 20 per cent of the world consume 80 per cent of its resources, and the wealth that the West currently enjoys (which allows us to use formula safely) was largely gained by colonising and plundering the very people from whom we feel so detached. In fact, our relatively comfortable lifestyles are built upon a system that controls markets through which poor countries provide us with cheap food, consumer products and labour. Our choices directly affect the lives of the people living in the wake of our consumption.

Western values have been influencing poorer cultures for centuries. For over 400 years, the expansion of colonial rule was a source of great pride. People in the West felt justified in using natural resources and cheap labour from other countries for profit in the name of progress. The colonies offered immense and irresistible new markets for Western goods and products. In the mid-20th century, the expansion of companies like Nestlé into these territories was swift and ruthless. They capitalised on exploitative and exclusive trade agreements to sweep in under the umbrella of imperious medical legitimacy. In *The Politics of Breastfeeding*, Gabrielle Palmer explains the effect that the introduction of formula had on these women: 'Many mothers were convinced that artificial milk was a sort of medicine, especially as it was endorsed and distributed through channels of health care.'[25]

> 'The companies who boasted about their ethical instruction "to be used only under the direction of a physician", in the US, abandoned this directive when they expanded their promotion into the Third World. They used every method they knew to persuade mothers to use their product: billboards, radio and newspaper advertising and "milk nurses" [...] Milk nurses were employed by the infant food companies to visit new mothers in the hospital or at home in order to sell them baby milk [...] They were usually paid on a commission basis and they earned more than any trained nurse in the health service [...] An investigation in Nigeria in the early 1970s showed that 87 per cent of mothers used artificial milk because they believed that they had been advised to do so by hospital staff who in reality had been milk nurses allowed into the hospital.'[26]

The introduction of the Western concept of timed feedings combined with poor working conditions that prevented mothers from taking their babies to work with them as they had always done in the past meant that women's milk supplies would quickly diminish. The 'need' for the substitute product was therefore magically created and the subsequent dilution of breastfeeding as a cultural norm became inevitable.

The 'milk nurses' of the 1970s may seem like ancient history, but today real nurses, who have grown up in a bottle-feeding culture, unwittingly promote formula as the right way to care for babies without even getting paid to do so. Formula companies have always worked hard to establish a relationship between their products and the medical professionals in whom we trust. They know it is a key element in the marketing machine. They sponsor events, target doctors, nurses and midwives with gifts and provide funding to build maternity units in hospitals all over the world. It is not a coincidence when these maternity units have separate wings for mothers and newborns, on different floors or on opposite sides of the hospital to one another. Separating mothers from their babies effectively guarantees that breastfeeding will not be straightforward, so this is a highly effective way of creating potential customers for the formula company associated with the hospital.

A July 2014 job description for a Nestlé post in Canada sets out the major responsibilities of the staff employed to target health workers (emphasis added):

» 'Stimulate retail sales through the promotion of infant formulas and cereals to **GAIN HEALTHCARE PROFESSIONALS' RECOMMENDATIONS** (physicians, nurses, etc.) based in community clinics and offices
» Manage and develop hospital accounts to targeted growth plan
» Prospect and **BUILD RELATIONSHIPS WITH TARGET HEALTHCARE PROFESSIONALS AND KEY OPINION LEADERS**
» Plan, lead and/or participate in medical education events/conferences'[27]

And in order to increase their presence within the UK healthcare system, Nestlé has set up a network of 'nutrition representatives' to target health workers. This is an extract from the job description:

'As Clinical Network Representative, your role is to work on the designated territory, visiting hospitals, doctors, health visitors and community midwives to develop key clinical relationships within your local health Economies, leading to opportunities for the SMA brand and Nestlé Nutrition [...] Working with the NHS at a territory level, you'll be developing long-term, mutually beneficial relationships with key stakeholders and opinion leaders to support brand endorsement and strategically aligned education for Healthcare Professionals.'[28]

This is in violation of the International Code of Marketing of Breastmilk Substitutes and clearly demonstrates how formula companies elbow their way in to favour with healthcare professionals. They know that there is no better way to gain brand loyalty than to get to us when we're in hospital. At a time when a mother is vulnerable, raw and needing to be cared for and shown what to do, it is easy to see why she might become strongly bonded to the brand of formula that she associates with the birth of her new baby.

Promoting formula to mothers in the UK might sound like fair game to some. No big deal. But the truth is that women and children in rich countries like ours are victims as well as beneficiaries of a capitalist system that prioritises growth above all else. Profit comes before people. But the wealth of capitalism *can* be put to good use. 'In 1970, breastfeeding rates in Norway were as low as those in Britain today. Then Norway banned all advertising of formula milk completely. They offered a year's maternity leave on 80% of pay and, on the mother's return to work, an hour's breastfeeding break every day. Today 98% of Norwegian women start out breastfeeding and 90% are still nursing four months later.'[29]

The situation in the UK is not quite so hopeful, but formula promotion actually threatens the lives of babies in other countries. In Bangladesh, Nestlé currently promotes infant formula with the claim that it is the 'gentle start' for babies. They informed their shareholders at a conference in 2015 that this marketing strategy would prove to be an 'engine for growth', which would seem to suggest that their aim is expansion rather than to meet an existing need. They had to change the wording of their campaign from a 'natural start', to a 'gentle start' following complaints by Baby Milk Action in October 2014. But regardless of the wording they use, their 'engine for growth' continues apace and their intentions are clear. 'A Save the Children survey in 2012 found health workers continued to report being targeted by company reps. with Nestlé most prominent.'[30]

In 2015, a film called *Tigers* was released which documented the true story of Syed Aamir Raza, a former Nestlé baby milk salesman, who turned against the company when he realised that babies were dying as a direct result of being fed formula rather than breastmilk. Far from being a David and Goliath tale of triumph, his campaign was crushed and he was forced to flee his home country and separate from his family following a series of anonymous threats and attempts on his life. Despite describing themselves as ambassadors for health, formula companies have never been troubled by a sense of responsibility for the lives of innocent people. Nestlé were aware that the lack of vitamin A in their sweetened condensed milk caused rickets, blindness and even death in babies who drank it as a breastmilk substitute, but they continued to market it as such until 1977, with the tagline 'the food par excellence for delicate infants'.[31]

VI) ALL IN GOOD TIME

For those mothers who do breastfeed, it can feel like there is a lot of pressure to wean a baby at a certain time, or at least not to let them become 'too attached' to the breast. The creation of follow-on milks by formula companies has further instilled in us the idea that breastmilk is not appropriate or necessary beyond the minimum recommended age for breastfeeding. It might be helpful to know that the World Health Organization and UNICEF recommendations on breastfeeding are as follows:

» Initiation of breastfeeding within the first hour after the birth
» Exclusive breastfeeding for the first six months
» Continued breastfeeding for two years or more, together with safe, nutritionally adequate, age appropriate, responsive complementary feeding starting in the sixth month [32]

However, many babies are not ready to start solids until later than six months and just because babies *can* be introduced to foods at six months does not mean that they are ready to start eating three square meals a day. Many a mother has noticed that the food she has lovingly prepared looks exactly the same on the way out of her baby as it did on the way in. Digestion is inefficient at such a young age and nutrients are less easily absorbed from solid or pureed foods than they are from milk. Babies do not have sufficient levels of the enzyme amylase (needed to digest starch from solid food) until they are around six months old, and it can take up to two years to reach mature levels. The carbohydrate enzymes maltase, isomaltase and sucrase do not reach adequate levels until a baby is around seven months old. Milk is much more nutritionally dense and easier for babies to digest than food, and breastmilk contains amylase to further assist digestion.[33] By giving a baby water with their food (which is necessary in order to prevent them becoming constipated), we are further diluting its nutritional value. Not only is this time-consuming, but it is counterproductive as well.

Many health professionals (and milk product manufacturers) state that after a year, cow's milk can be given to a baby instead of breastmilk, and one of the reasons cited for this is the need for additional iron. However, the iron in cow's milk is in a form that is not as easily absorbed by the baby's digestive system, meaning that he does not benefit from this 'extra' iron and might actually absorb less overall. Excess iron in the baby's intestine can also be a problem, because some bacteria feed off iron and can overpopulate the gut. The iron in breastmilk is bound to the proteins lactoferrin and transferrin, which means that this iron will only be available to the baby, preventing potentially harmful bacteria (such as *E. coli*, salmonella, clostridium, bacteroides, escherichia, staphylococcus) from using it to multiply.[34] Breastmilk also continues to support a child's developing neurological and immune systems throughout infancy, so although cow's milk becomes a feasible alternative to human milk after a year, it certainly does not become better than human milk. In the second year of a baby's life, 448 ml of breastmilk provides:

- » 94% of vitamin B12 requirements
- » 43% of protein requirements
- » 76% of folate requirements
- » 36% of calcium requirements
- » 75% of vitamin A requirements
- » 29% of energy requirements
- » 60% of vitamin C requirements[35]

There is a tendency in our culture to worry that children who are breastfed to term will never stop. We think of weaning as mother-led, rather than mutual – an obstacle to overcome – another job to do. But in many cultures, the winding-down of nursing is a natural progression like learning to walk and talk. The child's need for his mother diminishes and his wish to gain independence and join his older role models increases over time. Eventually, it just makes sense to let go and move on.

Jean Liedloff observed the natural succession of life stages over time among the South American Yequana tribespeople with whom she lived for many years. 'Living as one has evolved to do [...] Babyhood desires give way to those of the successive phases of childhood and each fulfilled set of desires gives way to the next.'[36] In this way, a person can grow up feeling at peace with himself and with the passing of his youth. He won't feel a sense of longing or regret unfulfilled needs. Liedloff knew that if you try to take something away from somebody before they are ready to let go, they will only resist more fiercely.

For those of us who do not live in the rainforest, the return to work is often a watershed in the nursing relationship. We worry about it for months in advance and it is often felt that the only answer is to work towards weaning. But in fact, by nine months, babies who are happy eating some solid food can drink water from a cup during the day, and will benefit hugely from the bonding and nurturing aspect of breastfeeding when their mothers return home in the evening. It can become a time to reconnect after a long day and share a joyful moment together.

There is no 'right' time to wean a baby from breastmilk. Various scientific studies have shown that, based on our size in relation to other primate species, the biological weaning age for humans could be anywhere between two and a half and seven years. The fact that breastmilk contains the perfect long-chain fatty acids for myelination of brain cells means that it would benefit human babies to continue to breastfeed while the bulk of this work is being done (which takes years, not months). It is also worth considering that it takes about six years for a child's immune system to mature fully.[37] Not only does breastmilk help to establish that immune system, but also provides some extra protection in the meantime. For these reasons, natural selection during our evolution might have favoured those babies who were breastfed for longer, meaning the instructions to breastfeed for the whole of infancy could be built into our genetic code.

Anthropologist Katherine Dettwyler reassures us that 'in societies where children are allowed to nurse "as long as they want" they usually self-wean, with no arguments or emotional trauma, between 3 and 4 years of age'.[38] The trouble is we have so few examples of this happening in our own experience that the idea seems very alien to us. But one mother who allowed her child to self-wean describes the moment it finally happened like this:

'Breastfeeding made mothering my younger child so easy, so simple, so wonderful. I was not strong enough to breastfeed my older one more than 6 months and I have never stopped regretting that [...] And his sister, aged four, came to me today to say goodbye to boobies. She said she is too big. She just stopped. She made this decision. Nobody demanded it from her. Nobody forced anything. Until today, nursing was the first thing we'd do in the morning and the last thing we'd do at night. It's hard for me to believe that it's over. More than four years and suddenly she doesn't want my milk any more. For the first time in her life she didn't ask for boobies to help her sleep. She has fallen asleep herself. Incredible. Maybe she will change her mind, I don't know. I am ready for this big change. I am so proud of us. We did it. Over four years.'[39]

In the end, we all have a choice, and many women choose to continue to breastfeed, often in secret, for longer than is generally deemed necessary or acceptable. I stopped breastfeeding my first child when I became pregnant with my second. All my energy was going into making the new baby and I could do no more than that. At the time my son was two and a half and I was able to explain to him why it was time to stop. It was a relatively easy transition, and involved very little resistance from him. By that time he was keen on the idea of being a big boy and not a baby. Other mothers make different choices for different reasons. The important thing to know is that though children do grow up and move on, breastmilk never stops being nutritionally beneficial. In some parts of the world, even adults are free to enjoy the benefits of human milk.

Ruth Kamnitzer lived in a traditional felt tent in the Mongolian countryside for three years while her husband, Steve, conducted a wildlife study. She describes the experience of breastfeeding her son, Calum, while living in Mongolia:

'When I breastfed in the park, grandmothers would regale me with tales of the dozen children they had fed. When I breastfed in the back of taxis, drivers would give me the thumbs-up in the rear-view mirror and assure me that Calum would grow up to be a great wrestler. When I walked through the market cradling my feeding son in my arms, vendors would make a space for me at their stalls and tell him to drink up. Instead of looking away, people would lean right in and kiss Calum on the cheek. If he popped off in response to the attention and left my streaming breast completely exposed, not a beat was missed. No one stared, no one looked away – they just laughed and wiped the milk off their noses.

'In Mongolia, breastfeeding isn't equated with dependence, and weaning isn't a finish line. They know their kids will grow up – in fact, the average Mongolian five-year-old is far more independent than [their] Western counterpart, breastfed or not. There's no rush to wean [...] the intervals between births are fairly long, most kids give up breastfeeding at between two and four years of age [...] But if weaning means never drinking breast milk again, then Mongolians are never truly weaned – and here's what surprised me most about breastfeeding in Mongolia. If a woman's breasts are engorged and her baby is not at hand, she will simply go around and ask a family member, of any age or sex, if they'd like a drink. Often a woman will express a bowlful for her husband as a treat, or leave some in the fridge for anyone to help themselves [...] The value of breast milk is so celebrated, so firmly entrenched in their culture, that it's not considered something that's only for babies. Breast milk is commonly used medicinally, given to the elderly as a cure-all, and used to treat eye infections.

'By Calum's second year, I had fully realized just how useful breastfeeding could be. Nothing gets a child to sleep as quickly, relieves the boredom of a long car journey as well, or calms a breaking storm as swiftly as a little warm milk from Mummy.'[40]

5. SLEEP: SAFE AND SOUND

Motherhood is about raising and celebrating the child you have, not the child you thought you'd have. It's about understanding he is exactly the person he is supposed to be. And, if you're lucky, he might be the teacher who turns you into the person you're supposed to be.

– Joan Ryan

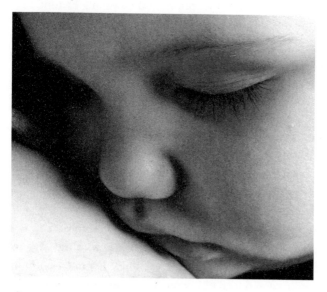

1) KEEP IT TOGETHER

There is a lot of talk about bad habits when it comes to bedtime and sleep. Children sleeping in bed with their parents is of course the main offender – the cardinal sin according to Western parenting convention. But what exactly are we so worried about? Creating clingy children? A disrupted sex life? SIDS? Child abuse? When we look closely at these issues it turns out that the significant factors involved are primarily social and environmental and have little or nothing to do with co-sleeping. Researchers are now finding proof, should any be needed, that humans are simply not meant to sleep alone and especially not in the fragile first years of life. The adult 'need' for babies and children to sleep alone is a relatively recent construction and one that is still largely confined to a handful of Western countries. Parents sharing their bed with their children is not a bad habit. It is normal throughout much of the world, and all of human history. On the contrary, I would argue that suppressing or misinterpreting our genuine emotional and physical needs is the bad habit of a lifetime. So why are we all doing it?

I was struck by this description of the evening routine in a farmhouse, in a remote region of Guatemala:

> 'Maria works hard but she is an unstressed, calm woman [...] Her children are polite and intelligent and take part cheerfully in the family subsistence duties: shutting up the pig and piglets at night, catching fish in the pond, shelling beans, making tortillas for every meal [...] During the evening after supper in the candlelit house, she cuddles her six-year-old son (her youngest and last child) until he falls asleep [...] all is peaceful.'[1]

Something about this passage resonated deeply in me. I came across it at a time when I was wrestling with the urge to keep my first baby with me in the evenings. I wanted nothing more than to sit and feed him while I watched TV, read a book, or talked through the day with my husband. But somehow, our baby's presence in the room felt like a failure, like something we should be ashamed of. At the end of a hard day, I desperately wanted the peaceful evenings that I imagined mothers like Maria enjoy. But I was repeatedly being told by those around me that I must wage war on my instincts and on my baby, in the name of an independence I did not want or need either of us to have.

After reading about more and more mothers like Maria, and realising that I was not alone in my feelings, I decided that my instincts were probably telling me what was best for our family after all. We stumbled onto the path of co-sleeping and have never looked back because life got a lot better when we did. Leading infant sleep researcher Dr James McKenna has noted, 'Parents with less rigid ideas about how and where their babies should sleep are generally much happier and far less likely to be disappointed when their children cannot perform the way they are "supposed to" – i.e. sleep through the night.'[2] Having waited for my baby to naturally learn to sleep alone, I can say that it was not an easy choice (and at times I wondered if he ever would), but he did, and I now have no doubts about my decisions. I'm sure most parents will tell you they made the right choice, whatever it was, and that is as it should be, as long as it was a genuine and informed one, but that is not always the case. It is heartbreaking to know that some mothers go along with the prevailing social current, only to find themselves regretful when they look back on things. This is the experience of one mother who has written very honestly about such feelings:

'My oldest came to my room after bedtime and said, "Caroline keeps saying she needs you." I went upstairs and looked at my sweet little one, who is now four, curled up under her covers peacefully. I said, "Do you need me?" She nodded. I knelt down, crawled into bed with her, and snuggled up close. "Lullaby, and goodnight [...]" I softly began to sing. I rubbed her head and nuzzled my nose into her hair, and felt the delicateness of her soft skin. She lay there precious and still, with heavy eyelids, and I kissed her head and thought, *How many times have I rushed bedtime? How many moments like this have I lost?* And it was there in her bed in that quiet moment that I realized how much she needed me, and how much I had neglected that need. When my straggly-haired hippie girl was only two-years old I did everything I could to get her to go to bed, but she wouldn't stay put. Sometimes she would get out of bed 20 times, and just about every time she would say, "I just want to be with you." I thought she was disobeying, and I felt like I was going crazy because I was so tired and I just wanted my own time; I needed a break. So after trying all sorts of discipline techniques, after crying, after praying, I would sometimes get angry and I took it out on that little girl just trying to figure out how to be with her mama. Because that's what it was about, she just needed me, maybe in bed with her, rubbing her head, singing to her, loving her; she just needed me to be with her. And all my fighting of it did nothing but cause pain and tears and regret.'[3]

My husband initially found it very difficult to accept my need to tend to our baby in the evenings. He thought, like so many of us, that it should be a time for adults, and that we were making a huge mistake by keeping him with us. He felt jealous and he was frightened of doing things that we were so strongly warned against. At times our difference of opinion seemed insurmountable and it pushed our relationship to the limit. Although I wasn't sure that I was right about what I was asking of him, he eventually began to realise exactly what it was *he* (and society in general) was asking of *me*. Upon my request he began to read about sleep in other cultures throughout history, and he gradually let go of some of his preconceived ideas. He actually began to think that what came naturally to me might be better for all of us, including him.

A couple of years later something happened at work that really affected him. He was marking some year one (six-year-old) school work for a project about night-time when he realised that almost every one of the children had written that they were afraid of the dark and didn't like sleeping. He told me that he couldn't believe how many of them had said in their work that they just wanted their mummy at night. Human infants are hugely adaptable and resilient, and this includes the ability to conceal unwelcome feelings in order to avoid the very worst outcome that they can conceive of: rejection and abandonment. So the very same impulse that makes them beg to be with their parents at night-time can prompt them to realise that it is better to accept what is out of their hands, and to stay in bed even if they are afraid. Their love and need for their parents' approval is at the heart of their actions, even when it appears otherwise.

Now that it is widely understood that human babies are essentially born three months premature, it has become socially

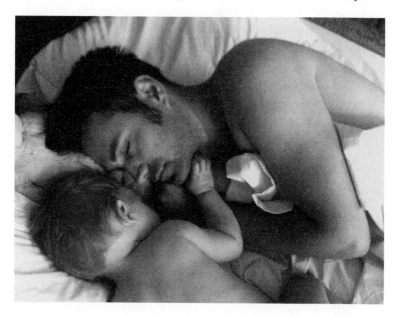

acceptable that they sleep near to us for the first three months, until they are out of the fourth trimester and in fact this is now recommended by UNICEF. But beyond this, it is still regarded as a mistake to allow a baby to become accustomed to sleeping in close proximity with adults. In Japan, it is not uncommon for children to sleep in the same room as their parents until they are young teenagers, at which point they naturally become keen on having their own space, but that idea is as foreign to us as the Japanese culture itself.

'The relationship between mother and child is viewed the same way by all – a baby is pure spirit, essentially good by design, and in need of being incorporated into the maternal self. Japanese babies and older children sleep between their parents to symbolise their position as a river between two banks, a being that is intimately connected to each parent as a river is to its riverbed.'[4]

In her book *Our Babies, Ourselves*, Meredith Small tells us, 'In almost all cultures around the globe today, babies sleep with an adult and children sleep with parents or other siblings [...] Mayans treat sleep as a social activity and think sleeping alone is a hardship.'[5] When approached by American researchers, who told them about the differences between the two cultures, '[t]hey expressed pity for the American babies who had to sleep alone. They saw their own sleep arrangements as part of a larger commitment to their children.'[6] We may look upon the customs of other cultures with consternation at times, but clearly it goes both ways. What is normal to us can be seen as alien and even ridiculous from a different perspective. While English mothers are often acutely aware of their babies' sleeping patterns, some Italian mothers would be unable to even answer the question. They typically sleep with their babies and do not keep track. However, if you ask them what their baby has eaten, they could talk about it for an hour.[7]

After several years living with Yequana Indians in the South American rainforest, Jean Liedloff's perspective on sleep was permanently altered. Of a baby's experience in a Western setting, she says:

'The things that are put within reach are meant to approximate what he is missing. Tradition dictates that toys be consoling to a grief-stricken infant. But it does so somehow without acknowledging the grief. First and foremost there is the teddy bear or similar soft doll "to sleep with". It is meant to give the infant a sense of constant companionship. The eventual fierce attachment to them that is sometimes formed is viewed as a charming bit of juvenile whimsy rather than a manifestation of acute deprivation in a child reduced to clinging to an inanimate object in its hunger for a companion who will not desert him.'[8]

Many paediatric sleep disorder experts strongly advocate the use of such comforters to settle babies. In his bestselling book *How to Solve Your Child's Sleep Problems*, Richard Ferber says '[t]he toy will often help him accept the night-time separation from you and can be a source of reassurance and comfort when he is alone [...] His toy will not get up and leave when he falls asleep and will still be there whenever he wakes.'[9] Ferber also warns us of the dangers of showing too much affection at night, because, 'if you always allow yourself to be used in the manner of such an object – to lie with him, or let him twirl your hair whenever he tries to fall asleep – he will never take on a transitional object, because he won't need to'.[10] In other words, he will be attached to you rather than to a toy. And what a disaster that would be.

In this passage, Ferber clearly identifies a child's need for comfort and reassurance while he sleeps, but fails to notice the inferiority of an inanimate object to another human being for a child's cognitive and social development. We have spent the past century short-sightedly trying to attach our children to objects rather than to people, and we have now reached the point where our tendency towards consumerism and materialism now threatens the very survival of life on earth. We have attached ourselves so strongly to our possessions that the thought of losing them is more terrifying than the possibility of our own annihilation.

Nevertheless, the words of such experts are taken as gospel by many parents and the importance of a bedtime routine appears to be sacrosanct. We are convinced that without this routine, our children will be unable to recognise the end of the day or even their own tiredness. 'American parents used lullabies, stories, special clothing, bathing and toys to ritualise the sleep experience, whereas Mayan parents simply let the baby fall asleep when they did.'[11] There is nothing wrong with an evening routine, but when we talk about it in our culture what we are describing is more like a schedule. A schedule is a series of things to be done at or during a specified time frame. A routine, on the other hand, is a natural rhythm that regulates the flow of the day, and it can accommodate any changes that arise. A schedule involves hitting time targets which is all about adults feeling that we are in control.

Babies need their parents to help them through the day. They need help to sit up, they need help to eat when they are hungry and to fall asleep when they are tired. They need to be talked to and cuddled and played with. They need to be gazed at and made to feel loved and wonderful. Sometimes at three o'clock in the morning they need to be carried up and down the hall until they feel sleepy again. I've done the 3am hallway walk and the 4am garden shuffle and the 5am 'okay never mind, let's just have breakfast' sigh. And I know that at that moment you're thinking, *But there MUST be a way around this!* And there is. And you will hear about it time and time again. And for many people it works. But there is no *right* way and there is no easy way. Sticking to a schedule and any form of sleep training is a lot of work. If I had a penny for every time I've heard someone say, 'We are working towards getting the baby to fall asleep by himself,' I'd be able to afford a night nanny (ha, only joking, kids). But to my mind, 'sleep' and 'work' just don't belong in the same sentence. So I take it as it comes and enjoy the cuddles while I can. Why not? They're only little once.

'Compared with the rest of the world, our parents do carry a huge amount of baggage about how terrible it will be dealing with an infant's sleep. Indeed, we are taught to expect an adversarial relationship with our babies (with regards to sleep) even before we meet them. Due to placing infants at odds with their emotions, i.e. socially isolating them for sleep, and/or minimising contact, which is exactly what infants seek and need, it is no surprise that Western parents (surely the most well-read and informed) nonetheless remain the most obsessed, judgmental, disappointed, exhausted and the least satisfied parents on the planet! I attribute much of this to the fact that the Western traditional infant sleep models and recommendations and conceptual expectations have always heretofore been determined by social ideologies, social "wish lists", having little to do with who babies are biologically, preferring instead to define infant needs in terms of who we want them to become and notions as to how, for example, to make them "independent" at young ages and, thus, we create the very sleep environments and unrealistic parental expectations that create and perpetuate the very sleep "problems" sleep "experts" are asked to solve.'[12]

II) BREAK IT UP

Jean Liedloff marvelled at the relaxed attitudes towards sleep that the Yequana people of South America seemed to have. In *The Continuum Concept*, she recounts how easily they slipped in and out of sleep and how sleeping lightly was not seen as a problem. She recalls:

> 'Their habit of telling a joke in the middle of the night, when everyone was asleep. Though some were snoring loudly, all would awaken instantly, laugh and in seconds resume sleep, snoring and all. They did not feel that being awake was more unpleasant than being asleep, and they awoke fully alert, as when a distant pack of dangerous peccary was heard by all the Indians simultaneously, though they had been asleep.'[13]

Perhaps our perception of sleep as sacred, and our need for sleep to be undisturbed is more about our lifestyle than our babies. The tribespeople that Liedloff describes were free to nap during the day, and could sleep as many or as few hours at night as they chose. They had a tendency to wake early in the mornings, but it was not a beeping alarm that roused them. In contrast, it is the fact that sleep feels like a rare commodity to us that makes it seem so precious. The industrial society that we have created imposes pressures on our time that aren't compatible with relaxed attitudes towards sleep. But there are people for whom the eight-hour block of sleep is meaningless.

The !Kung San of Botswana think nothing of waking up in the middle of the night. They will happily spend a few hours around the campfire talking, singing and socialising. They allow for a natural break in their sleep to tend the fire, the animals and the children. There is no notion of insomnia in their culture, because no one is expected to sleep solidly through the night.[14] And there was a time when it was not so different for us. Our babies appear to know something that we have all forgotten. We in the West also used to have two sleeps during the night.

I remember often having to get up at 5am with my wakeful baby. While my husband slept soundly, I paced the floor with him, eyes aching, feeling cheated and resentful, waiting for his little body to surrender to sleep again, so that we could go back to bed. One morning as I peered through the curtains, I saw that it was snowing outside. The flurries whisked around street lamps and swirled around trees and my gaze drifted across the road, to the house opposite. They also had a young baby, and I sometimes took comfort in seeing that their lights were on at all hours of the night. The loneliness is always the worst part of being up early with a baby. Eventually he dropped off again and we went back to bed, but when we woke again, the snow had gone. Nobody else I spoke to that day knew that it had snowed. I realised then that those moments with my baby were special. Quiet, lonely, but somehow tender, I managed to cherish these quiet hours when I had my second baby because I knew they wouldn't last for ever. The night-time needs of our babies are fleeting and bittersweet, just like a flurry of snow before dawn.

Looking over to see if your neighbour's lights are on might sound insignificant, but there was a time when it would not have

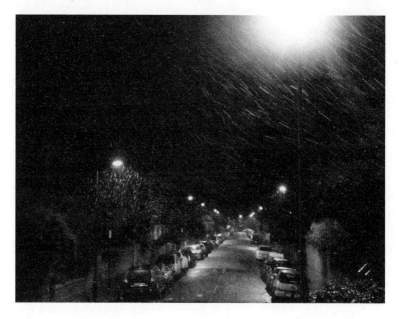

been unusual to go and pay your neighbour a visit if you saw a light on in the middle of the night. History has all but forgotten that a few hundred years ago we took our sleep in two four-hour blocks, separated by a period of quiet nocturnal activity. When we lived by candle light, people typically retired to sleep a couple of hours after sunset. They would then have two sleeps and the hours in between were used to go to the toilet, eat or drink something, read or write, chat to loved ones, tend to infants, and have sex. A doctor's manual from 16th-century France advised that the best time to conceive a child was not at the end of a long day's labour 'but "after the first sleep", when couples might "have more enjoyment" and "do it better".'[15]

As well as expressing their devotion to one another in between sleeps, many people also used this time to express their devotion to God. Prayer books from the late 15th century included specific prayers for the hours in between sleeps.[16] It was such an accepted part of ordinary life, that no one bothered to document it. All historical mention of the 'two sleeps' is purely incidental, which may be why it was able to fall out of common knowledge as our society changed.

It seems incredible that this has been forgotten, especially since cultures that sleep in this way are still in existence. There is evidence that this is a very natural way for humans to take their rest. Psychiatrist Thomas Wehr conducted an experiment in the early 1990s, which sought to answer the question of what sleeping pattern is natural for humans. A group of people were subjected to darkness for 14 hours a day for a month. 'It took some time for their sleep to regulate, but by the fourth week the subjects had settled into a very distinct rhythm. They slept first for four hours, then woke for one or two hours before falling into a second four-hour sleep.'[17]

So why do we now sleep all in one go? The answer revolves around the Industrial Revolution and the changes that took place once street lighting became commonplace. Before 1684, cities were dark and dangerous places at night, but the introduction of street lighting meant that you could stay out late in relative safety. 'Nightlife' changed from being the quiet time you spent with your family in between sleeps, to an exciting extension of the day, which could be continued indefinitely or until you were too tired to carry on. The Industrial Revolution also brought with it changes to our working patterns. Factories required employees to spend a block of time during the day working intensively away from home. The hours available for rest in between became restricted and precious. Eventually our sleeping pattern began to mirror our working day. Efficient and productive, we got the job done. By the 1920s the two sleeps had become a thing of the past. But babies, who are unable to go long stretches without food, toilet and reassurance, didn't adapt so easily and the 20th-century obsession with 'problematic' infant sleep was born.

III) THE SCIENCE BIT

Biological anthropologist and leading sleep researcher, James McKenna does not believe that infant sleep is inherently problematic. His studies have shown that babies sleep in a way that is biologically appropriate and even protective for them. Having first specialised in the social behaviour of monkeys and apes, he began to apply the principles of behavioural evolution to human infants after the birth of his own son in 1978. He was recruited to the University of Notre Dame in 1997 where he studied the way that mothers and babies sleep, both together and when separated.[18] Like all sleep experts, he observed behaviour, but McKenna went a step further and developed techniques for recording brain activity, heartbeat, breathing and sleep stages (REM sleep vs. deep sleep). He discovered that mothers and babies who sleep together will synchronise, and regulate one another's bodies. A mother's sleep pattern automatically changes to adapt to the needs of the baby, and she can respond without consciously waking. Crucially, the baby is stimulated by the mother's breathing, helping him to recover from sleep apnoea (pauses). This is important because these short pauses in breathing are thought to sometimes cause sudden infant death syndrome (now sometimes called sudden unexpected death in infants, or SUDI).

As a result of this evidence, the doctor responsible for spearheading sudden infant death syndrome (SIDS) funding and education in America since the 1970s is now calling for doctors to stop saying that co-sleeping is dangerous. Abraham B. Bergman, the first president of the National SIDS Foundation, wrote an editorial for *JAMA Pediatrics* (published by the American Medical Association) in 2013 entitled 'Bed Sharing Per Se Is Not Dangerous'. In it he calls out the American Academy of Pediatrics for making unfounded claims against bed-sharing with babies, and calls for consistency in how infant deaths are classified.[19] This is because the death of a baby from SIDS will often be recorded as related to co-sleeping in any instance where the baby was not sleeping alone in a cot. If an exhausted mother falls asleep on a sofa or chair with her baby and it becomes trapped and suffocates, that might well be recorded as a co-sleeping death.

In fact, almost all instances of SIDS actually occur in the presence of other contributing factors that have nothing to do with bed-sharing. Alcohol or narcotic consumption, obesity or unsafe bedding are often the real culprits when a baby dies in his parents' bed. Making co-sleeping taboo has actually made it dangerous. Parents who only do it occasionally, when they are very tired or when the baby is ill, are less able to make sound judgements regarding safety. It's so easy to fall asleep on the sofa, or forget to reduce the clothing and bedding covering the baby (our body heat keeps babies warm and overheating is a major risk factor).[20]

What parents need is information, so that we can address the risks and make better decisions. We get plenty of advice about using a cot safely (place the baby on his back with feet at the foot of the cot; don't let him get too hot or too cold; don't fill the cot with toys; keep blankets away from his face; no pillows, etc., etc.). These guidelines just go to show that using a cot involves risk too, after all, SIDS used to be called cot death. Care must be taken when co-sleeping, but the message given to parents is *don't do it* and for many this is simply unrealistic. We are told we should breastfeed our babies, but co-sleeping, which is an important aspect in many breastfeeding relationships, is a no-no. The 'guilty secret' stigma that now surrounds it has cut off the conversation and babies pay the price. In fact, there is evidence to suggest that sleeping with our babies, especially if we are breastfeeding, is actually *protective* against SIDS when done in a safe, considered way.

'[The] human infant is the most vulnerable, contact dependent, slowest developing and most dependent primate-mammal of all, largely because humans are born neurologically premature, relative to other primate mammals [...] This means that its physiological systems are unable to function optimally without contact with the mother's body, which continues to regulate the baby much like it did during gestation [...] This is a profoundly true scientific beginning point to understand why babies will never accept nor respond to the memo that says they should sleep alone. The solitary infant sleep environment represents a neurobiological crisis for the human newborn as this micro-environment is ecologically invalid for meeting the fundamental needs of human infants. Indeed, sleeping alone in a room by itself and not breastfeeding are now recognized as independent risk factors for SIDS, a fact that explains why most of the world [has] never heard of SIDS.'[21]

The United States has the highest rate of SIDS on the planet. It is the single greatest cause of infant death in a country where GDP is consistently higher than any other. I have heard it said that people in other cultures would surely put their babies in separate rooms if they had enough money to do so, but that would certainly not prevent deaths from SIDS. McKenna despairs:

'I worry about the message being given unfairly (if not immorally) to mothers; that is, no matter who you are, or what you do, your sleeping body is no more than an inert potential lethal weapon against which neither you nor your infant has any control. If this were true, none of us humans would be here today to have this discussion because the only reason why we survived is because our ancestral mothers slept alongside us and breastfed us through the night!'[22]

McKenna has theorised that the moderate increase in the level of CO_2 in the immediate vicinity of a co-sleeping mother and child acts as a respiratory stimulant that triggers the baby's brain to react in the event of a breathing lapse.[23] This, combined with other sensory stimuli like the smells, sounds and movements of his mother, improves an infant's chances of avoiding or recovering from breathing errors during sleep. It gives his brain opportunities to refine its breathing regulation controls.

McKenna's studies have also revealed that infants who sleep alongside their mothers experience 'less deep sleep, shorter bouts of [dangerous] deep sleep, more frequent arousals, significantly increased breastfeeding sessions, but also more total sleep when in their mother's presence than when sleeping alone'.[24] Many mothers would argue that they put their babies in separate rooms precisely to ensure these longer, deeper sleep periods, believing that deep sleep is better sleep, for both them and their babies. But it is important for babies to practise transitioning through sleep stages and not to get 'stuck' in deep sleep for too long. Mothers who co-sleep from the start may experience more frequent waking, but they may be able to manage them more smoothly without having to leave the bed. And those who co-sleep from the beginning often learn to sleep through slight interruptions or return to sleep quickly without waking fully.

'When McKenna scored mothers' co-sleeping behaviours and compared them to what mothers did when they slept in a different room and got up at night to attend the baby, co-sleeping mothers exhibited five times the protective behaviours toward their babies. They repeatedly kissed, touched and repositioned the baby. They readjusted blankets and comforted the baby when it fretted. And sometimes these mothers, as the polygraph showed, were not even conscious.'[25]

Because of this, people often worry that parents will become so used to co-sleeping that they might roll over and squash the baby. Anthropologist Meredith Small categorically dismisses this argument: 'Western parents who fear they will suffocate babies are wrong. In a healthy atmosphere, where parents are not intoxicated, on drugs or obese, the chance of killing an infant by overlaying is zero.'[26] Even if the mother is confident that she will not roll over onto her baby, many believe that the father poses a threat. While precautions can be taken within the sleeping arrangement to protect against any potential risk, research at the University of Notre Dame has shown that fathers show lowered levels of testosterone while co-sleeping, compared to those who do not. This suggests that they are also biologically adapted to sleep in a protective way with vulnerable infants.[27] It would be reasonable to conclude then that it is more dangerous to co-sleep occasionally when a child is upset or ill than to do it consistently, because these protective adaptations may not be triggered in the parents.

A fear of squashing babies in our sleep originates from events deep in our past. In medieval times, infant deaths were often reported as being due to 'overlaying', and this got to the point where laws were enacted in most European countries to prevent parents from sleeping with their babies.[28] But all was not as it seemed. In a time before contraception and when food was scarce, there would be a pressing need for peasant families to limit the number of hungry mouths to feed. It was not uncommon for babies to be stifled in their sleep and for the death to be called an accident. Essentially these laws were passed as a means of preventing infanticide, but the association with co-sleeping and smothering has stuck.[29]

Babies who co-sleep often sleep on their side for some of the night while breastfeeding, and there is a strong case for the idea that not only is co-sleeping protective against SIDS, but that it is better for physical development too. By spending time in different positions, the baby's soft skeleton is not subjected to extremes of pressure for any length of time. This means that the back of the skull, the spine and ribcage are less likely to become flattened, and the hips and legs are less likely to become splayed. (You can now buy 'sleep-nests', which are designed to combat the problems caused by the supine sleeping position.) It is also thought that this flattening may contribute to delayed motor skills. In traditional cultures like the !Kung San, 'the baby is always positioned vertically [because] babies left in a horizontal position will never develop good motor skills, they believe'.[30] And this belief is supported by the fact that !Kung San babies do surpass their European peers, typically developing the ability to walk competently and unaided somewhere between nine and 11 months.

IV) TRAINER DANGER

There is no such thing as a baby...
A baby cannot exist alone, but is essentially part of a relationship.
– Donald Winnicott

There is an elegant symbiosis between a sleeping mother and her child. McKenna's research shows that 'mothers and infants experienced simultaneous brainwave changes often within seconds of one another, and sometimes without any overt behavioral change'.[31] Sleeping side by side tunes our bodies in to one another without us even realising it. Our baby starts to take cues from us about how sleep works and how to regulate it, as he gradually progresses towards sleeping for longer stretches. And we receive the information we need from him too, allowing us to respond better to his needs.

But conventional wisdom in the West states the very opposite. We are told we must teach him by removing ourselves and imposing unnatural conditions on him. We want it done as quickly as possible and we see the end result as the primary goal, but we are asking a lot and perhaps we are missing the bigger picture. We are told we can expect our baby to sleep independently at three months old, and yet a three-year-old is not expected to be able to cut food with a knife, climb up high to reach something, or control his own bowels. But with all these things, if a child is allowed the opportunity to develop his skills gradually, without pressure, he will become adept and confident in his own time. Children are all about *the process*. Trying to short-cut anything will result in resistance. And I do mean anything. As adults we usually have a goal in our mind whenever we do anything, but that is meaningless to our children. They experience love and learning through the time we spend allowing a process to unfold.

Although many 'baby whisperers' promote gentle methods, the voices of their predecessors still haunt us. And gentle or not, the ultimate goal of sleep training is still independence and consolidated, solitary sleep. But surely therein lies a contradiction. Typically anything that involves training creates individuals who accept dictation and do as they are told. But the true spirit of independence is thinking for yourself and trusting your intuition. It just doesn't add up.

Like any new parent, James McKenna turned to the words of sleep experts for advice when his own time as a father came, but he was quick to see that their wisdom was flawed:

> '[A]fter reading a few books about how best to care for your new baby we were left with one of two conclusions: either everything we had learned in anthropology, my specialty, was wrong, or all these Western recommendations about how best to care for babies had nothing to do with babies at all. Maybe it had everything to do with recent Western cultural ideologies and social values that more accurately reflect what we want babies to become, rather than who they actually are and what they need.'[32]

The preaching of such experts – paediatricians, domestic goddesses and baby whisperers – weighs heavily on the shelves of bookshops and libraries, and the minds of uncertain parents.

They offer lengthy prescriptions that they claim will 'cure' a dysfunctional baby and return peace and harmony to a household. The author of one recent title includes advice about *scheduling cuddles at particular times of day*. (Yes, you read that right). She also warns that when practising sleep training, it is important to be strong-willed should your baby cry to the point of vomiting, because it is only a ploy to manipulate you. She advocates changing the sheets quickly and efficiently without comforting, picking up the baby or even making eye contact – lest you might give him hope. It's not what any of us signed up for when we decided to have a baby, but the pressure to get him sleeping through the night is immense and we find ourselves doing things we never dreamed we would have to.

The pages that contain these hard-line doctrines are invariably nestled beside pictures of healthy, happy babies – full of the promise of perfection and success. These books are a literary wolf in sheep's clothing. One technique in particular has achieved remarkable popularity (or notoriety, depending on who you ask) over the past 30 years, despite its ruthless approach. The Ferber method, devised by Dr Richard Ferber, advocates leaving a baby as young as five months old to cry unattended for up to 45 minutes. Many people swear by his method's effectiveness, and I have no doubt that for those with the stomach to follow it through there may be a good night's sleep to be had. But this achievement becomes hollow in the face of evidence that solitary sleep contradicts the biological imperatives for healthy emotional and physical development.

The Ferber method, like most extinction sleep techniques, relies on the fact that eventually a baby will realise he cannot effect change in his circumstances (or 'get what he wants') when he cries, and will simply stop trying. For some infants this may be unpleasant, but tolerable. For other more sensitive souls, this feeling of abandonment can have severe consequences. Under the ominous title 'Other Problems', the penultimate chapter of Ferber's book, unlucky number 13, covers the subject of head-banging, body rocking and head rolling. Just to be clear, this chapter is not about developmentally challenged children. According to Ferber, repetitious rhythmic behaviour around sleeping is normal. He describes babies rocking on all fours, rolling their head from side to side, banging their head against the headboard or dropping it down repeatedly onto the pillow or mattress.

He states that these 'normal' rhythmic behaviours are not observed from birth and usually emerge around six months of age – soon after he says sleep training can begin, funnily enough. They typically escalate towards head-banging and head rolling by about nine months, but he reassures the reader that it rarely continues beyond three or four years of age (perhaps because these children are no longer confined to their cots by then).

Astonishingly, he romanticises this behaviour, claiming that it may be soothing, and he compares it to an adult swaying to soft music.[33] He does admit that it is not clear why a child would find this type of repeated impact comforting, when an adult would not. Perhaps Ferber had never been to the zoo and seen wild animals pacing in their cages when he did his research. When restrictive conditions and social and sensory deprivation are imposed upon a sentient being, head rocking is quite a common response.

Ferber is a father and a doctor and unfortunately these credentials are enough to convince parents that he knows better than they do. The good doctor's book came out in 1986 and it boasted about the six years of research that went into it, but in 1999 Ferber recanted his own words about the importance of solitary sleep for a child's development. 'I wish I hadn't written those sentences [...] That came out of some of the existing literature. It is a blanket statement that is just not right. There are plenty of examples of co-sleeping where it works out just fine. My feeling now is that children can sleep with or without their parents. What's really important is that the parents work out what they want to do.'[34] Ferber sounds contrite on the subject, but his book is still available to buy, and enjoys five-star reader reviews, with enthusiastic comments like 'It works!'. Perhaps it does, but for how long, and at what cost? Sleep training often has to be repeated over and over again during a child's early development, and the effects are not immediately obvious.

In her book *Why Love Matters*, psychoanalytic psychotherapist Sue Gerhardt says, '[O]ur earliest experiences as babies have much more relevance to our adult selves than many of us realise. It is as babies that we first feel and learn what to do with our feelings.'[35] Babies are born with only 25 per cent of their eventual brain mass, but it is not simply the case that the brain must become bigger and better. Significant sections of the brain simply do not exist during infancy and have to be built from scratch. Gerhardt says, '[W]hat needs to be written in neon letters lit up against the night sky is that the orbitofrontal cortex, which is so much about being human, develops almost entirely postnatally [...] [so] it is no good trying to "discipline" a baby or to expect a baby to control its behaviour, since the brain capacity to do so does not yet exist.'[36] The idea that a fretful baby can learn to self-soothe is therefore a complete myth. All he can really do is learn to give up or play dead.

Unfortunately, the nature of human brain development is such that the times when a baby demands attention the most may be the times when his parents will be tempted to deny him it, fearing that they will spoil him. The brain develops in bursts rather than steadily progressing, and new layers of perception are rather abruptly bolted on to the existing ones. Experiencing one of these bursts can be troubling for some babies. It's like going to sleep with the world in black-and-white, and waking up to it in technicolour. Babies can become cranky, clingy and difficult during these developmental leaps, and often find it hard to settle for sleep. Parents may be sympathetic when their baby is getting a new tooth, because it is clear to see the cause of the upset, but a new level of brain development is invisible until after it has happened, so unless you know what's going on, you could be forgiven for thinking that stronger discipline was needed. Fortunately, some very clever scientists have mapped these leaps and we can now predict precisely when one is going to happen (see chapter 7).

The orbitofrontal cortex is part of the cerebral cortex (the thinking brain), which is the final layer of the human brain to develop and a later evolutionary addition to the limbic 'mammalian' brain. The orbitofrontal cortex regulates the primitive impulses which originate in the 'reptilian' brain stem. Strong emotions like rage, fear or sexual desire are generated in these primitive subcortical regions, but are monitored by the orbitofrontal cortex, which will intervene to prevent inappropriate behaviour. '[O]rbital and adjacent cortices are [...] critically involved in decision making and behavioral choice.'[37] Brain scans have revealed that Romanian orphans who were severely neglected and left alone in their cots for long periods of time had massively underdeveloped orbitofrontal cortices. The same was found to be true of a large proportion of criminals when their brains were scanned.[38] These two examples point to the conclusion that deprivation of positive human contact inhibits development in the orbitofrontal cortex and that the result may be an impaired ability to regulate antisocial impulses.

Sleep training is used as a means of teaching independence and self-ownership, but to Gerhardt this argument does not stand up. 'Unfortunately, leaving a baby to cry or to cope by himself for more than a very short period usually has the reverse effect: it undermines the baby's confidence in the parent and in the world.'[39] Attuned and attentive care, on the other hand, generates opiates in the baby's brain, which not only feel good but actually facilitate the growth of the medial prefrontal cortex.[40] And poor development of this area of the brain during infancy is linked with depression later on in life.[41]

Many mothers feel that withdrawing attention and affection is acceptable if it is only done at night. But removing emotional caregiving for 50 per cent of a baby's life, and especially during the hours when the brain is assimilating and consolidating information, may impact the baby's development in a way that ultimately compromises his ability to regulate his emotions. Gerhardt describes how in depressed adults there is 'a reduced density of neurons in the dorsolateral part of the prefrontal cortex, the area that develops in toddlerhood and is involved in verbalising feelings'.[42] This means that fewer neurotransmitters like serotonin or norepinephrine are released, which help to regulate and improve mood. It also means that such individuals will be less able to judge situations and control their reactions appropriately in order to manage stress.[43]

There has also been a lot of research into the effects of stress on a baby's brain. The stress response is triggered when a baby finds he needs something but cannot attain it. If his attempts to communicate are met with an inappropriate or inadequate response, his only options are to cry louder or withdraw mentally.[44] In either case a cascade of chemical reactions are triggered by the hypothalamus which result in the release of cortisol.

Cortisol is the emergency response hormone that communicates with the rest of the body in an attempt to manage a crisis. It tells the body to shut down nonessential systems such as immune function, growth and learning.[45] Not only does this inhibit the baby's immediate physical and emotional development, but as Gerhardt explains, '[T]he kinds of emotional experience that the baby has with his caregivers are "biologically embedded". They get written into the child's physiology because this is the period of human life when regulatory habits are being formed.'[46] Cortisol exposure is toxic to the developing hippocampus, preventing it from forming and functioning properly. The hippocampus is in charge of informing the hypothalamus when it is time to switch off cortisol releasing factor (CRF), so if it does not function properly, it inhibits the feedback system which regulates the stress response. This means that the brain can easily become flooded with cortisol, with no ability to switch it off.[47]

This early imbalance can result in prolonged and poorly regulated periods of stress, anger and depression in adult life. It has been shown that among women co-sleeping during childhood is associated with less discomfort about physical contact and affection as adults. The same study showed that boys who co-slept with their parents between birth and five years of age had significantly higher self-esteem and experienced less guilt and anxiety.[48] Another study showed that co-sleeping appears to promote confidence, self-esteem and intimacy.[49] But, on the other hand, a UK study showed that among children who never slept in their parents' bed, there was a trend to be harder to control, less happy, exhibit a greater number of tantrums and to be more fearful than children who slept in their parents' bed all night.[50]

When a baby's brain is developing, it is continually storing experiences along with the corresponding automatic responses, by creating new neural pathways. When experiences are repeated, those pathways are strengthened and will eventually become myelinated or 'sealed in' permanently. This happens when myelin, a protective, fatty sheath, is laid down to insulate a new neurone. The neural pathways that are created in response to experiences which are *not* repeated will *not* be reinforced in this way and so these unused pathways will eventually wither and be 'pruned' away. This explains why infants can recover extremely well from trauma. But it also means that the more consistently a negative experience is repeated the more likely it is that it will permanently affect the brain's eventual response patterns.[51]

Much is made of the idea that a baby can and should learn to 'self-soothe'. This phrase has become the trusted mantra of baby whisperers everywhere and fills the hearts of desperate parents with hope. But the whole concept is based on a myth. According to researcher Dr Thomas Anders, who invented the term in the 1970s, it was never anything more than an expression used in their experimental literature to describe a baby who settled himself back to sleep without signalling to his parents (that is, a 'self-soother'). It was not originally intended to be used to describe any skill or ability that could or should be learnt or taught. He says:

> 'Self-soothing is a label we coined to contrast with signaling (crying) upon awakening. I would bet that most non-signaling awakenings occur without active self-soothing [...] [W]e chose the terms "signaled" awakenings vs. "self-soothing" awakenings. The latter term was meant to imply a developmental trajectory on the road to self-regulation.'[52]

So the original use of the term was simply to label those babies who were not distressed upon awakening, and who naturally returned to sleep. Self-soothing was never considered an optimal or better behaviour, just one of two options. The trouble with scientific jargon is that it can be taken out of context and misinterpreted. From the moment it is out in the world, it has a life of its own and can be used to legitimise false claims.

The other thing about sleep training which sticks in my throat is that such 'methods' can become a commodity for sale. Whether you buy a book or you pay for a private consultation, the experts are making a living by perpetuating the idea that something needs to be done, to be fixed – that the problem lies with the baby, and not with our expectations. The fact that babies do naturally progress towards consolidated sleep has been written out of the equation. Arbitrary deadlines are set for sleeping through the night, and we believe in the idea that not only does it have to happen quickly, but that it has to be parent-led if it is to happen at all. As a society we are complicit in a system that creates increasingly restrictive parameters for our sleep to fit into. Our language is littered with phrases like 'get back to work', 'don't be caught napping' and 'no sleeping on the job'. We blame babies for our lack of sleep, without noticing that it is we who have created a world that does not allow for it.

The idea that better sleep can be secured in return for

money is deeply entrenched. We invest our money and our hopes in sleep strategies, baby monitors, swaddles, sleep suits, comforters, pacifiers, sound and light machines and blackout blinds. There is no end to the number of products that promise to make it all better. But guess what? The best baby monitor on the planet is a human being. Nothing will ever trump parental attentiveness and intuition. Children grow up and stop needing our help to fall asleep in their own time. By 18 months my first son, who was a 'terrible sleeper', no longer needed a wee at night, and at two and a half he started sleeping solidly through the night, from around 8.30pm until 6.30am without stirring for milk. I often wondered how long it would take, but ironically, by the time it happened I no longer felt a desperate need for uninterrupted sleep. At three years old he was so relaxed about bedtime, that he started climbing into bed and kissing the sheets, the pillow, the bed frame, and saying, 'I love the bed.' He would then be happy to lie down and close his eyes without any ritual or persuasion. He knew he was safe and valued there.

As I type, I have a sleeping toddler nestled in my lap. The day is done and he is snoring gently. When he chuckles in his sleep, I wonder what tickles him in his dreams. I look forward to these precious moments, when this crazy ball of energy gets all soft and dreamy and sleepy in my arms. I know now that it all happens naturally, and I'm content being able to say with certainty that he did it in his own time. I'm off to bed soon, and I'll be carrying him up with me. After a lot of soul-searching, I don't feel bad about that any more. The proof is in the pudding, and this little pudding is delicious.

If you focus on the positive, believing firmly that your baby is exactly as he should be, accepting that his needs are legitimate, and his potential infinite, then your response to these needs can be an opportunity for bonding, trust and confidence to flourish. Fear and resentment can evaporate and everyone can relax. That's not to say that you will suddenly have a really easy baby on your hands; some babies just have a lot going on, but you will have ensured a positive dynamic between you for the future of your relationship. If you show your baby respect from the very start, he will understand that as the correct way to behave. He will learn to trust you and himself, which is perhaps the greatest gift that you can offer a child.

After everything we have covered in this chapter (and at the risk of conforming to the feminine cliché of apologetic self-justification), here are my personal reasons for choosing to co-sleep until my children are ready to move on:

» My first baby did not want to sleep alone. (If he had slept well in a cot, I would have put him in one. I didn't know anything about brain development then and we certainly did try to 'make it work'.)

» I don't think bedtime should be a battle. The thought of struggling with my children when we are all tired and need to rest in order to get them to conform to someone else's ideology doesn't make much sense to me.

» I don't like the thought of bed-hopping. It just doesn't seem conducive to rest, so we decided to pick a location and stick with it. All of us. All night.

» I don't want my children to fear the dark or dread bedtime. Sleep is such an essential and significant aspect of our lives, I think it's worth starting out with a healthy, positive attitude towards it.

» I like co-sleeping. I like feeling my children's warmth and hearing their breath; knowing at any given moment that they are comfortable and safe helps me enjoy my sleep too. I love hearing them chuckle in their sleep, and the first crazy things that come out of their mouths when they wake up.

» My babies like it. Why should I deny simple pleasures to the ones I love the most? Pleasure should not become tangled up with guilt.

» It gives us all more time in bed.

» I can put my baby on a potty when he needs to wee in the

night. This builds trust and communication between us. My eldest was out of nappies at night by 18 months and my youngest by six months. I kid you not. (See chapter 8.)

» The bed is big enough. We are tall so we have a super king-sized bed, which is wide as well as long. We struggle when we go away and have to sleep in a double or queen-sized bed, so I understand that space can be an obstacle. In that case, an open-sided cot (at the same level and without a gap) next to the bed is one possible solution.

» When my second baby arrived, his older brother stayed in the big bed with us. It was a way to stop him from feeling pushed out. It was clear to him that he had not lost his place and I think it helped.

» Somehow I felt sure that my children would want their own space one day, so I stopped worrying about when that day would come. Everyone says, 'They grow up fast,' and they do.

However, there is no such thing as a free lunch, as they say, and the drawbacks to co-sleeping include:

» Finding yourself sleeping in awkward positions and having to roll over ooohh soooo slooooowlyyyyy.

» Sleeping in a cardigan because you can't pull the covers up past your waist.

» Tiny flailing limbs that result in blows to your face and upper body.

» Occasionally waking to find there are little feet on your head.

» The bed is no longer the epicentre of your sex life, which is an opportunity to find imaginative solutions. As the saying goes, where there's a will, there's a way.

» The general dismay, disbelief and disapproval of everyone you know.

» Feeling the need to write a book to justify your actions.

6. STRONG FOUNDATIONS

If you were the ocean, I'd be the sand.
If you were a song, I'd be the band.
– J.J. Heller

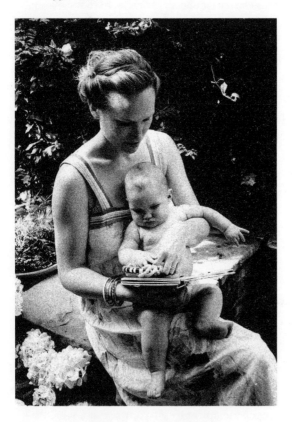

I) ABOUT ATTACHMENT

Respectful, responsive, instinctive parenting is no longer the preserve of hippies and nonconformists. It has now become a legitimate brand of parenting with a name: Attachment Parenting, or AP for short. It stems from the work of Mary Ainsworth and

John Bowlby about attachment theory, but it is the American doctor William Sears who neatly packaged it up and promoted it to the mainstream as an acceptable 'alternative' choice. Emerging as something of a backlash against the prevailing wind of authoritarianism in Western childcare methods, AP now jostles for position alongside the big guns in the modern day melange of parenting styles. But the 'brand' can be off-putting. After all, most parents dare not risk acquiring a label that might invite judgement, criticism or even rejection by others at a time when we need all the help and support we can get.

AP is essentially nothing new, but it is often portrayed as if it were by the controversy-hungry media. To some extent the problem lays in the word 'attachment' which for some might portend the creation of a possessive, grasping or 'clingy' personality. I don't think the name does the AP movement any favours. Bonding is also a key aspect of AP practices and this can be taken the wrong way too. Bonding may be critical to the development of good parent–child relationships, but to be bonded (shackled?) to someone sounds a teeny bit worrying. And if the mother and child are 'bonded' together, where does that leave everyone else in the family? Attachment Parenting seems to invoke suspicion and many people are quick to dismiss it entirely. But when I had my babies I was relieved to discover a childcare literature that was willing to say 'go with your gut'. The AP approach does come with a set of principles, but rather than feeling I had to follow them to the letter, they gave me courage and confidence in my ability to find my own way.

The Seven Bs of Attachment Parenting are:

» Birth bonding
» Breastfeeding
» Bedding close to baby
» Baby-wearing
» Belief in your baby's cries
» Beware of baby trainers
» Balance

Going with your gut sounds straightforward enough, but it's not a habit we're really into. We're so used to problem-solving that it can be tricky knowing our gut from our grey matter. AP requires a leap of faith. It's hard to find examples of 'where it all might lead'. Damn those hippy children for turning out normal and blending into society. And when we're newcomers to the school of parenting, doing the wrong thing is a terrifying prospect. Everything seems to hinge on starting out on the right track and people are full of talk about not spoiling your child, not making a rod for your own back, and what *might* happen if you don't push for long-term goals as early as possible.

Everyone seems to believe that children who are 'indulged' with respect and kindness will never grow up, that they might sleep in your bed for ever or breastfeed indefinitely, and never learn to function independently. Mulling over these woeful prophesies, it gradually occurred to me that these are *not my fears*. I worried that my children would grow up disconnected from their own emotions, or with no one that they feel they can trust. I worried that they might grow to feel inexplicably angry, lonely or insecure, like so many of the adults I know. It turns out that all the advice about encouraging independence (or detachment) didn't reflect my priorities anyway. In fact, it sounded to me like it might just be causing some of the things that I feared the most.

I was curious how things turn out for families who choose not to conform and I wondered what happens when whole societies do things differently. Could there be a correlation between peaceful parenting practices and peaceful cultures? Psychologist Robin Grille thinks so: 'Authoritarian or harshly patriarchal child rearing can incline any nation or ethnic group towards violence.'[1] Barbara Nicholson and Lysa Parker agree: 'Numerous scientists and leaders have long believed that the parent–child relationship holds the key to the very survival of humanity; some believe it is the key to world peace. We call the type of parenting these scientists have observed in peaceful cultures around the world attachment parenting.'[2] As former UN secretary general Kofi Annan once said, 'Much of the next millennium can be seen in how we care for our children today.'[3] If Kofi said it, you know it must be true.

Michel Odent also points out that peaceful parenting starts from the very first moments of life. Respect granted to the critical bonding period immediately after birth between mother and baby affects a society as a whole. He says, '[A] simple conclusion can be drawn from a rapid overview of the data we have at our disposal: [t]he greater the social need for aggression and an ability to destroy life, the more intrusive the rituals and beliefs are in the period surrounding birth.'[4] Essentially, we can look at cultures throughout history and around the world and observe the correlation between respectful parenting and egalitarian societies.

Robin Grille has studied the history of violence around the world. In his book *Parenting for a Peaceful World*, he concludes that 'the most positive social changes around the world have followed mass improvements in the way in which children are treated'.[5] He goes on to say,

'For humans, the bridge between instinct and behaviour is built by our learning experiences. Early life experiences mould our raw aggression, determining whether it will manifest as rage and hostility; or as creativity, innovation, industriousness and leadership [...] [C]omparative studies among European nations have found strong links between harsher child-rearing modes and increased levels of civil or cross-border armed conflict, delays in democratic reforms, and greater public resistance to the responsibilities associated with democratic freedoms.'[6]

The essential thread that runs through everything attachment parenting stands for is *connection*. Connection is about listening and it's about trust. The quality of the connection between individuals is the key to the whole deal – from relationships within families, communities and societies, all the way up to the global community – the warp and weft of human connections that spreads across the entire planet. We evolved to live in extended families, and we are nourished by positive connections, not bound by them. Trust and respect are natural by-products of a strong connection and they eliminate the need for systems of control to promote peace, because when we feel heard and understood, there need be no resentment within us. People who feel that no one listens to them get angry, and angry people lash out.

II) THE ROOTS GO DEEP

The human brain and heart that are primarily met with empathy in the critical early years cannot and will not grow to choose a violent or selfish life.
– Robin Grille

The roots of attachment parenting go way back to the beginnings of human history. Many AP practices like co-sleeping, breastfeeding and carrying babies in a sling are essentially very primitive. But ironically, modern science is 'discovering' that these basic principles are still appropriate for human infant care, and that they might actually promote optimal development. In the mid-20th century, psychiatrists Mary Ainsworth and John Bowlby began to recognise the significance of emotional health, and how early life experiences related to this, when they traced the sources of their patients' emotional and behavioural problems back to childhood trauma and, in particular, to separation and abuse.

Bowlby theorised that early experiences of abandonment could directly affect the development of the brain, leaving not just haunting memories, but an indelible difference in the structure and function of our most vital organ. He made a connection between strong parent–child attachments and robust mental health and this established the framework for the theory of attachment.

> '[A] system [within the brain] controlling such behaviour as attachment can in certain circumstances be rendered either temporarily or permanently incapable of being activated [...] What are being excluded in these pathological conditions are the signals [...] that would activate their attachment behaviour and that would enable them both to love and to experience being loved.'[7]

Brief periods of stress or trauma in life are inevitable, and perhaps even necessary, so the question for psychiatrists became: where do the boundaries lie, and what constitutes *irrevocable trauma*? In the years since Bowlby's original hypotheses, a great deal of research has been done in this field and it is now believed that experiences during the critical period of development in the first four years of life dictate the physical shape and function of the brain. So the emotional life of an individual can be determined by early childhood experiences. According to Bowlby, the keys to attachment are proximity and responsiveness. This may seem obvious, but it is these two things that are often actively discouraged by many baby experts even today. In Bowlby's words:

> 'There now seems little doubt that when infants and young children are the subjects of insensitive mothering, mixed perhaps with occasions of outright rejection, and later to separations and threats of separation the effects are deplorable. Such experiences greatly increase a child's fear of losing his mother, increase his demands for her presence and also his anger at her absences, and may also lead him to despair of ever having a secure and loving relationship with anyone.'[8]

Bowlby observed the results of poor attachments in patients who had experienced neglect, but Jean Liedloff, the author of *The Continuum Concept*, studied a very different set of individuals. Living among indigenous South American tribespeople, she saw how babies, who clung to their mothers for much of their first year, became increasingly bold in their explorations. With time they naturally ventured further afield, and were trusted to not only return when they were ready, but to test the limits of their own abilities and to judge for themselves when their safety was in question. 'In general his first expeditions are short and cautious and there is almost no need for his mother or caretaker to take a hand in his activities. Like all little animals, he has a keen talent for self-preservation and a realistic sense of his capabilities.'[9] Venturing out on his own terms allows the child to develop a strong sense of himself. His mother trusts him, so he feels he can and must trust himself too.

Liedloff and Bowlby both conclude that securely attached babies take longer 'excursions' away from their primary caregiver over time, proving that it is not necessary to push a child into independence. 'By eight months of age almost every infant observed who had had a stable mother figure to whom to become attached showed this behaviour; but, should the mother be absent, such organised excursions became much less evident or ceased.'[10] Bowlby also states that it is human nature to require a secure base throughout our lives, even into adulthood. Seen like this, 'dependency' is not a sign of abnormality or weakness in an infant, and contrary to popular belief, forcible detachment from the primary caregiver could be more likely to cause clinginess than prevent it.

Children don't learn independence. They grow independent. And they do it naturally in their own time, just like they learn to crawl and walk and talk in their own time. The simplest and most effective approach to growing independence is, ironically, to meet children's attachment needs. It is trust that frees children to grow, explore, and develop, not forced independence or broken attachments.

– L.R. Knost

How the child experiences their world is what counts towards their emotional development, not what adults believe to be in their best interests. If the infant feels abandoned, even if they are left with someone the parent knows to be caring and competent, the experience is still traumatic, and this is potentially damaging. In *Why Love Matters*, psychoanalytic psychotherapist Sue Gerhardt explains that in order to express our love for our children in a way that is emotionally and developmentally nourishing to them, it is important that we think about our actions from their point of view. It is quite possible that, in the course of attempting to prepare them for the harsh realities of life, we could disrupt the development of their nervous system.

'[S]ituations that are unpredictable, which take you unawares, which you want to resist but have little power to change, are defining characteristics of stress. From this point of view, it is clear that babyhood can be extremely stressful without the support of tender, protective parenting.'[11]

Gerhardt goes on to say that raising an infant's stress level – such as by consistently ignoring him when he cries – won't teach him how to deal with it better, rather it could be damaging because 'high levels of cortisol in the early months of life can also affect the development of other neurotransmitter systems whose pathways are still being established'.[12]

My father-in-law was genuinely baffled that my eight-week-old baby should cry when strapped into a car seat. What he perhaps couldn't see was that *being* safe and *feeling* safe are not the same thing. It really depends on your perspective. It's a tricky issue to navigate if you want to follow the path of attachment parenting because parent–child separation is built into practically every aspect of our lives. We are divided by invisible lines that put children in separate boxes, 'safely' tucked away from the 'real' world, the adult world. But it doesn't have to be like that. In Argentina, 'even single and childless folks don't seem to think of little ones as a drag in many group settings. On the contrary, they believe children add a certain lightness, humour, and even hope.'[13] And '[i]n Buenos Aires, even if a child has a fit in a public place, almost no one glares. In fact, fellow customers, waiters or restaurant owners might come over and help.'[14]

In the UK we tend to orchestrate 'age-appropriate' events for children, away from disapproving glances. It is strangely difficult to find places to go that satisfy the needs of both adults and children. I found I didn't actually enjoy singing nursery rhymes in a circle of other mums I didn't know. The only thing that felt nourishing *for me* about the playgroups we went to was the tea and biscuits and even that was a guilty pleasure. Rarely am I able to take my children with me to the places that I want to go to. Even when space is made for children within 'adult' settings, it seems always to have been an afterthought and it is usually separated by some kind of physical barrier or dividing line. Play areas are often small (presumably because children are small), with no natural light and filled with grubby plastic imitations of adult objects to play with. 'The Garden' at the Science Museum in London is a sensory play area designed especially for preschoolers. It sounds lovely until you go there and find out that it is actually a dark, cramped room loaded with plastic 'educational' play equipment in the basement of the building, next to some toilets. You couldn't design a space more likely to induce a meltdown if you tried. Children need space and natural light. They need to move and play and interact among people of all ages, to be involved, included and integrated so that they can learn appropriate behaviour and be at ease in adult company.

Children desperately crave the company of their parents and they want to be a part of their society, but they are not invited to the adult party. All too often their presence is at odds with their environment. They're too lively, too clumsy, too messy. They have to be on best behaviour, because they don't fit in. They idolise older role models and virtually all forms of play mimic what adults do, but they are continuously cast out and condescended. And then they grow up to reject the adults who rejected them. Sitting in a cafe my three-year-old once said to me, 'It's really sad that everything in here is for grown-ups.' He was almost right. There was a separate play area for children with a miniature table and chairs tucked away in a cupboard under the stairs. But I couldn't sit in there with him and funnily enough, that's not where he wanted to be.

III) PUT THAT BABY DOWN

You should never let your fears prevent you
from doing what you know is right.
– Aung San Suu Kyi

As baby trainers love telling us, a baby is essentially manipulative. But when you consider that manipulation is his primary means of survival, this sounds perfectly reasonable. It is neither good nor bad, just necessary. He is asking us to care for him because he is unable to care for himself. And one of his primary needs, alongside being fed and kept clean is to be touched. Physical contact with another human being is vitally important to him. The warmth and strength of human touch allows him to feel safe, to relax and to flourish.

Like all primates, humans go through a complex bonding process. In the early 1980s, we learnt that babies release endorphins during the birth process, so for a certain time following birth, mother and baby are impregnated with opiates. The property of opiates to induce states of dependency is well known, so it is easy to see how this might facilitate the beginning of a dependency – or attachment – between mother and baby. Bowlby observes that 'the most significant variable predicting differences in maternal bonding was the length of time a mother had been separated from her baby during the hours and days after his birth'.[15] Close proximity in the first hours after birth certainly gets bonding off to a good start, but a degree of initial separation can be tolerated, because unlike other animals that imprint at birth or not at all, the human bond establishes gradually. In fact, it's perfectly normal *not* to fall deeply in love with your baby at first sight (especially if you had a traumatic birth or are in an unsettling environment), which is an encouraging thought for those of us who expected to feel something that we didn't.

A foster parent can become strongly bonded with another's child, and it seems that species that live in sophisticated social groups, like humans, typically form lots of cross-connections between individuals over time. This allows for cohesion, harmony and cooperation to prevail, which is just as well, because it definitely takes more than two hands to raise a human baby. As I said before, it takes a village to raise a child, and it's built into a baby's DNA to expect an abundance of eager arms waiting for him.

Efé pygmies are considered to be one of the oldest peoples still alive on earth, and it is thought that their way of life has changed little throughout the millennia. Living in the rainforests of the Congo in Africa, an Efé infant will spend 50 per cent of his time with someone other than his mother during the first four months of his life, interacting with around five adults per hour. Children typically constitute only a quarter to a third of the population, and nearly half of women have either one child or no children at all during their lifetime, so there are plenty of extra pairs of hands, and the children have many maternal figures other than their birth mother to enjoy.[16] 'In a social system that values community above all else, this multifaceted bond produces a tight network of social relationships.'[17]

It's not until you find yourself caring for a baby 24 hours a day, and alone for much of that time, that you begin to mourn for something that you never knew was gone. The Village of our ancient ancestral past is lost. In the UK, even people who live in villages often live lonely lives, separated by walls, fences and personal differences. The loss of the Village is something that has quietly taken place over centuries. We were so preoccupied with building and buying things that we lost sight of something we really needed. Increasing expectations for personal space and the arrival of technologies that do the work of many hands meant that we shut our doors and looked inwards. The nuclear family was born and the Village was lost. The strong, supportive web of family and friends that would have once been there to catch new parents has been allowed to become thin and blow away, just like an old cobweb. Caring for children can be hard, lonely work. You look around to see who can hold the baby while you go to the loo, and find there is no one there. You take pictures of the funny thing the baby did and post them online because there is no one there to share it with. You look back and realise you know the words to a dozen nursery rhymes, but you didn't know that your favourite band released a new record. Two years ago. You need company, but everyone is busy. You google local play groups. As Jean Liedloff says, 'A woman left alone every day with her children is deprived of social stimulation and needs emotional and intellectual support they cannot give.'[18] In fact, it can be harmful not only to her, but also her children, the rest of the family, and even society itself:

'[a] parent whose day is centred on childcare is not only likely to be bored, and boring to others, but is also likely to be giving an unwholesome kind of care. A baby's need is to be in the midst of an active person's life, in constant physical contact and stimulated by a great deal of the kind of experience in which he or she will take part later in life.'[19]

John Bowlby also laments the loss of community:

'[L]ooking after babies and young children is no job for a single person [...] [T]he caregiver herself (or himself) needs a great deal of assistance [...] In most societies throughout the world these facts have been, and still are, taken for granted and the society organized accordingly. Paradoxically it has taken the world's richest societies to ignore these basic facts. Man and woman power devoted to the production of material goods counts a plus in all our economic indices. Man and woman power devoted to the production of happy, healthy and self-reliant children in their own homes does not count at all. We have created a topsy-turvy world.'[20]

We talk a lot about our needs outside of our children. The need for time alone, for time with friends, for time to pursue our interests or our careers. We say, 'You can't fill another's cup if yours is empty,' which is absolutely true. In Western culture, the answer appears to be to get back to work. This solution immediately answers the need for adult community and allows parents to continue to develop their own interests outside their child. Yet for those who choose to stay at home with their children, the feeling of being undervalued, undersupported and excluded from the realm of economic productivity can be crippling. If we choose the path of attachment parenting, there is a tendency for people to sign us off as having martyred ourselves. It is as though we have revoked our rights to enjoy other interests or relationships with other adults – even our right to admit to feelings of isolation or abandonment by our peers.

As it stands, although many parents never report their feelings, it is estimated that between 10 and 20 per cent of women in the UK suffer from some from of perinatal mental distress or disturbance that is so severe they seek help from a doctor. Unfortunately, the top-down dynamic of seeking help from professionals that is often our only real option is part of the bigger picture of disempowerment for ordinary folk. Even when help is available in a crisis, the truth is that on the whole mothers aren't getting the kind of support that we need. Many of us arrive at parenthood only to find that the material dreams and aspirations that we have been trained to value offer no support when every day we are faced with the prospect of spending 10 hours alone with a baby. We need a physical, palpable social support network. Hand-to-hand. Face-to-face. Heart-to-heart. A Village.

The extended network of the Village is not just good for parents. Babies yearn for the hubbub of being outdoors and surrounded by the ambient hum of a busy community. It helps them settle, it helps them sleep. And although older children can usually cope with life in a nuclear family, they are generally not well adapted to it either. Too much time indoors and too few playmates mean they become frustrated by unmet needs that they can't verbalise. All they can do is express discontentment, which is interpreted as ungratefulness, insolence or deviance. One woman cannot hope to satisfy the social needs of her children 24 hours a day, no matter how much play dough she makes, how much Lego she builds, or how many play dates she arranges. In the Village, a child would have his pick of playmates, teachers and role models. Time with others and time alone would become a matter for personal choice, rather than running in accordance with school or working hours. Adults and children of all ages could mix freely, providing a rich tapestry of experiences and interactions throughout the day.

'Traditionally in many places from the Polynesian Islands and Kipsigis farms in Kenya to *villaggios* in Italy, diversion – as well as teaching and discipline – is a responsibility that belongs to other children [...] A vivid example of this can be found in the Polynesian Islands, where the idea of *whanau*, or wider family care, prevails. In those intimate communities, everyone – including extended family and neighbours – pitches in to help care for children, but there is a heavy reliance on siblings and peers for socialization and play.'[21]

But this is undoubtedly a dying way of life, and like it or not, we must adapt to the world in which we find ourselves. Romanticising about how things should be or used to be only gets us so far. We have to be resourceful in fulfilling the needs of our babies in the Western context. One of the central tenets of attachment parenting is that of strapping babies on and carrying them. This allows the parent or carer to go about our day in a manageable way with our hands free for other children, not to mention cooking, cleaning and going to the loo. But it also delivers the appropriate care for the baby. In his early days, a tightly wrapped sling secures him in a womb-like embrace. He can hear your heartbeat and feel your breath. He feels secure and safe, and many babies who won't nap well in a crib will happily go for long stretches in a sling.

As a baby gets older, being in the sling gives him a view of the world from a secure base. He can still retreat into sleep when he needs to, but he gets to feel he is a part of the adult world, safe, but not separate from it.

'Besides food and warmth, nothing is more important to your infant than snuggling close to you during the first four months of her life. As long as she experiences lots of physical contact, her development will not be delayed, even if you don't have much opportunity to play with her. A young baby generally loves lying close to you and being carried around. At the same time, this is a good opportunity for her to learn to control her body.'[22]

Carrying a baby upright also ensures his core muscles and

inner ear are stimulated correctly for their development.[23] This means that his strength, motor skills and sense of balance are refined with every step we take. It also addresses the problem of 'baby-container syndrome', which is a phenomenon whereby a baby's head becomes flattened or his neck favours one side to the other. This can result from spending too much time on his back and in cots, loungers, buggies and car seats. An American study observed 'a fivefold increase in posterior plagiocephaly [flattened head] comparing 1990–1992 with 1992–1994, and all infants, retrospectively, were found to be supine sleepers'.[24] These dramatic results were attributed to the introduction of new recommendations by the American Academy of Pediatrics in 1992 on the safest way for babies to be put to sleep in a cot. The campaign was a great success in that it reduced the incidence of SIDS by more than 40 per cent, but the malformation of babies' skulls as a result was an unexpected and perplexing consequence. A 'baby container lifestyle' has also been blamed for an increase in the number of babies experiencing motor delays.[25] 'Supine-sleeping infants showed delayed motor milestones in gross motor movements requiring upper body strength (roll, sit, pull to stand) in comparison to a prone-sleeping group.'[26]

Although this delay usually corrects itself once babies start to be able to move around a bit more, it feels like we are heading down the wrong path with the way we are handling our children. Indeed the answer to the problem from many paediatricians appears to be to lay babies down on their tummies during waking hours instead of their backs. 'Aim for three hours of "tummy time" per day by the time your child is two months old,' suggests one physical therapist.[27] This sounds painfully unrealistic to me as there are few babies who would enjoy three minutes of 'tummy time' let alone three hours, but this approach seems also to be missing a vital point: babies simply shouldn't be left lying around. In rural African communities, where babies are constantly carried upright and encouraged onto their feet as soon as possible, they will often develop motor skills like sitting, standing and walking earlier than European babies.[28] It's not a race to get to walking, and perhaps it doesn't matter how long it takes, but it makes me wonder about the wisdom of putting babies down on their backs all the time, and it supports the idea that upright carrying is a good way to go.

Ironically, the term 'baby container' would at one time

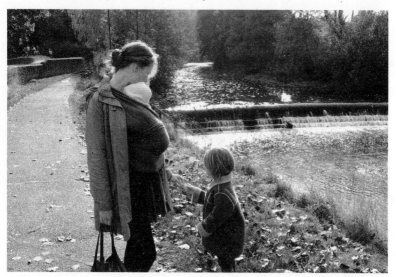

have meant some form of swaddle, sling or basket. There are images of babies in slings in ancient Egyptian artwork and the variety of different carrying methods across cultures is vast. But the trend to put babies in pushchairs is relatively new. In 1733, the Duke of Devonshire commissioned William Kent to construct a means for parading his children around as a novelty. He built a highly ornate shell-like basket on wheels that could be pulled along by a goat or small pony. Queen Victoria hugely popularised perambulators (prams) by having her children taken out in them, and in the 20th century the folding pushchair became established as an essential modern parenting aid.

Before this revolution took place, a baby who could not yet walk was called a 'babe in arms' because that's where he would usually be. Today, many babies are lucky if they clock up a couple of hours a day being carried, or even in physical contact with another human being. Carrying babies is a lost art and the loss of the term 'babe in arms' reflects a cultural shift which means babies are now seen as a burden when carried. In Britain, today it is widely considered 'right' that a baby be put down or put in something whenever possible. People often seem surprised to see me carrying my baby in a sling and I'm often asked, 'Isn't he heavy? Doesn't your back hurt?' and the classic question: 'Do you ever put him down?' The answers are yes, no and yes, of course I put him down. But why are people so perplexed? I would undoubtedly be congratulated if I was spending time 'getting back into shape' at the gym or training for a marathon. To pursue fitness for the purpose of wearing tight jeans or achieving personal goals is fine, but becoming strong in order to fulfil your child's needs is perceived as extreme, unnecessary or even weird. Why is that?

Some babies may be perfectly happy in a buggy, but others (like mine, for example) will protest, especially when they are very young, so for me the sling was the obvious answer. It is the feeling of security that the sling offers which is so appealing to newborns. Ina May Gaskin says that touch is the first language we speak. 'What a mother communicates to her baby when she holds him with a good firm touch is that he can relax; she's not going to drop him – it's all covered.'[29] And this is where baby-wearing and attachment parenting come together. Although the 'attachment' starts off very literal and quite intense, with time it becomes less physical and develops into a more general feeling of emotional security and trust.

A newborn baby draws a wealth of information about his world from touch. His other senses are muddled, and the warmth and scent that come from human flesh tell him he is safe. Buggy straps may tell his parents that he is safe, but they mean nothing to him. His brain is not even capable of perceiving himself as a separate being. Swimming in a sort of sensory soup, he cannot distinguish between his body and the world around him. Young babies see themselves as an extension of the person caring for them and when that person is removed, it can be disorientating and even frightening.[30] Many parents can accept this idea in the very early days, but after a few months, it's sometimes harder to understand why a baby can't yet cope with periods of separation. Unfortunately, as he grows to realise that he is a separate person, he may become even more frightened. He understands his own vulnerability and helplessness more than ever, and he is right to be worried. What could he possibly do to save himself if he were in danger?

While babies may have any number of reasons for feeling frightened or unsettled, there is really only one thing they can do about it. The sound of a baby crying is at once heartbreaking and infuriating, especially if we can't understand the problem. It can often be tempting to conclude that there is no problem, or that he is just crying for attention. But whatever the problem is, and whatever the solution may be, one of the most important messages from attachment parenting is to believe that our babies are attempting to communicate with us through crying. Crying is the precursor to a more sophisticated form of communication, and often babies who cry long and loud turn out to be chatty children. It is his voice for the time being, and he needs to feel that someone is listening and that what he says matters to us.

The work of Mary Ainsworth suggests that 'infants whose mothers have responded sensitively to their signals during the first year of life not only cry less during the second half of that year than do the babies of less responsive mothers but are more willing to fall in with their parent's wishes'.[31] When we respond to a baby, even if we feel that it is pointless, the eventual pay-off is a child who knows that his voice and his problems matter to us, no matter what. The common accusation that responsive parents will allow their children to dominate them once they are older overlooks the reality that when babies are responded to appropriately and taught that feelings matter the result can be a child who learns empathy and an ability to cooperate without the need for threats or bribery. It is a slow process, but worth believing in because, as Bowlby explains, human infants 'are pre-programmed to develop in a socially co-operative way; whether they do so or not turns in high degree on how they are treated'.[32]

And it is our culture that dictates the way children are treated, so it is sometimes hard to discern what is healthy or 'right' and what is not. No one could argue that the customs of ancient or tribal societies were always more baby-friendly than our own. Quite the opposite, because cruelty towards children has been rife throughout history. We must be selective about where we look for positive models to draw from and build upon.

Jean Liedloff described how humans are innately social. She realised that it is in our interests to conform to our culture as a means of survival, and babies and children are programmed to survive. Her observations of the Yequana tribe convinced her that on the whole we grow to behave in the way that our culture *expects* us to, not the way it *instructs* us to. She was amazed that the Yequana adults had no perception of children as unruly. Exuberance was accepted as part of a child's nature, and unacceptable behaviour was corrected. But children were never told that they were wrong or bad, only that their actions were incorrect. As a result, they felt no resentment and the tribe was cooperative and cohesive. Liedloff says that the children 'were uniformly well behaved: they never fought, were never punished, always obeyed happily and instantly'.[33]

> '[W]hat really matters is whether the parent meets those temperamental inclinations with the kind of response that the baby needs, and whether the parent is able to establish a reliable, loving relationship with that baby which can become the foundation for later social discipline [...] This child is less likely to need socialisation through fear and punishments because he is beginning to grasp the effect of

his own actions on other people and to be aware of their feelings. This happens only because his adult carers have been responsive to his feelings in the past and have convinced him that relationships are a source of pleasure and comfort, and therefore worth preserving.'[34]

Hold your baby. Listen to your baby. Trust your baby. Trust yourself.

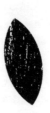

7. TWO STEPS FORWARD, ONE STEP BACK

Just because you can't see it doesn't mean it isn't there. You can't see the future, yet you know it will come; you can't see the air, yet you continue to breathe.
– Claire London

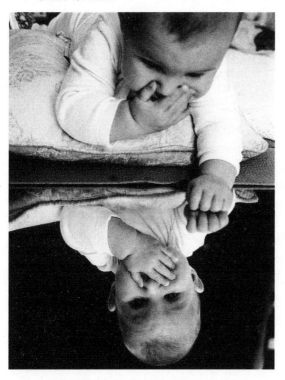

I) THE HUNGRY CATERPILLAR

It will come as no surprise to hear that babies grow in bursts. It seems to happen overnight. I have found myself reaching for the same Babygro my baby was wearing a week before, only to find it's now stretching at the seams. We marvel at how a baby can have a hungry phase one week and then his buttons will be bursting open the next. But we don't always think of brain development like this. It is easy to assume that a steady accumulation of knowledge, experience and repetition add up to a baby reaching his mental milestones. But in fact his brain grows in sudden bursts just like his little arms and legs do.

A baby's brain undergoes a series of rapid transformations which occur roughly every six weeks or so, with a gap in between for consolidating new skills. And each time this happens, he will seem suddenly different from the baby he was before. He will be doing clever new things, seemingly out of nowhere, and although every baby is different, all babies' brains are built up in a sequential way, one thing after the next. They literally can't run before they can walk.

Every new parent spends the first six weeks of their baby's life waiting for those first glorious smiles. We are hoping they will come sooner rather than later, but the truth is, we know that we have to wait. There are sleep-smiles and wind-smiles and half-smiles. But we always know a true smile of recognition when we see it. The prize is tantalising, but it comes at its right time and not before. Certain things have to happen in a baby's brain to get him to the point of producing a smile. It happens in a sudden rush of changes at around five weeks of age, and this is the first in a whole series of developmental 'leaps'.

We may revel in these wonderful changes, but it is all easier said than done for a baby. Shifting a gear in his level of perception is quite an ordeal, so much like the hungry phase before a growth spurt, he might have a fussy phase before a brain burst. The change itself will seem to have happened overnight, but the fussy phase can last for days or even weeks while the groundwork is being laid. Like the eventual appearance of a new tooth or the start of a cold, the reason for all the fuss sometimes only emerges after the fussy phase has passed. The older the baby gets the more complex the changes become and the longer the fussy phase can be. He'll have had a leap forward, but you won't know about it until after the storm has cleared and the dust has settled.

For some babies, this new layer of consciousness takes some getting used to. Like Dorothy in *The Wizard of Oz*, he finds himself caught in a twister and when he wakes up, the world is in stereo sound and technicolour. It's exciting, but also overwhelming. His mood may be unpredictable during the transition so he could be bursting with enthusiasm one minute and then inexplicably cranky, clingy or tearful the next. His horizons have expanded, but he can't get there yet and he doesn't know why, so he's frustrated and he will probably lose sleep over it. Like a butterfly emerging from a chrysalis, he comes out the other side of his 'leap' with amazing new abilities, but the metamorphosis can be quite an ordeal for him and he needs a little help.

'When her world has been turned inside out, she will be completely bewildered. She will cry, sometimes incessantly, and she will like nothing better than to be simply carried in your arms all day long. As she gets older, she will do anything to stay near you. Sometimes she will cling to you and hold on for dear life. She may want to be treated like a tiny baby again. These are all signs that she is in need of comfort and security [...] Because your baby senses something changing, she feels insecure and has a greater need for close skin-to-skin contact [...] Give her all the cuddling she needs and all the contact you feel you can handle at times like these. She needs time to adjust to these new changes and grow into her new world. She's accustomed to your body scent, warmth, voice and touch. With you she will relax a little and feel contented again. You can provide the tender loving care she really needs during this trying period.'[1]

The scientists who discovered these leaps were a Dutch couple called Hetty van de Rijt and Frans Plooij. They had been studying the development of chimpanzee infants and recognised a pattern whereby the chimps' levels of ability would graduate in sudden bursts. Van de Rijt and Plooij's findings were supported by existing work on hierarchical perceptual control theory (PCT) and they found that the pattern they uncovered could be applied to every species of primate they observed. They were curious to see if the same was true of humans and sure enough, after 35 years of observation, they concluded that it was.

They plotted the chart of human brain development and found that babies' brains make leaps forward at the same point after conception. Moreover, no matter what extra help and encouragement their parents offer them, the building blocks for certain abilities are simply not there before the corresponding leap has happened. Once these building blocks are in place, it is then up to the child and his carers to utilise them in order to develop those skills. Nature first, nurture second. For example, no baby can learn to grasp a toy before he has gone through the fourth leap, which starts at around 14 weeks and lasts about eight weeks. He just won't have the right bits in his brain to do it. But after that point, other factors like aptitude, practice and active encouragement determine how quickly he will master the skill.

Van de Rijt and Plooij argued that while the degree to which the changes affect a baby will vary, 'we are now able to predict, almost to the week, when parents can expect their babies to go through one of these fussy phases'.[2] And though the leaps are very pronounced in babies, they don't stop there. Van de Rijt and Plooij theorised that leaps continue to occur throughout life, with major ones taking place during the teenage years. It is important to remember that *they begin from conception and not from birth*.[3] The brain is built up in layers, starting with the primitive reptilian brain (the brain stem), which develops early on in pregnancy, and culminating with the formation of the uniquely human cerebral cortex. With every new layer added comes greater complexity as the brain becomes increasingly 'human'. Because of this, a baby's birth date can be misleading when anticipating the changes ahead. If he is born before or after his estimated date of delivery, it will affect the timing of his leaps, so babies cannot be compared to one another according to their birth age. This is perhaps one reason why the leaps are not immediately obvious, but there is no doubt that once you know one is coming, it makes the experience a lot less stressful.

'Often mothers think that there is something wrong with their tiny screamers. They think that she's in pain, or that she may be suffering from some abnormality or disorder that has gone undetected until now. Others worry that the milk supply from breastfeeding alone is not sufficient. This is because the baby seems to crave the breast constantly and is always hungry. Some mothers take their babies to doctors for checkups. Of course, most babies are pronounced perfectly healthy and the mothers are sent home to worry alone.'[4]

(Of course, whenever you think your baby is ill, whether during an anticipated leap or not, don't hesitate to seek medical advice.)

Aside from the fussy phases (which can be torturous for everyone), one of the hardest challenges that the leaps present to parents is to adapt quickly to the change. Just like a growth spurt calls for a step up in clothes size, it is out with the old and in with the new when it comes to the type of interaction he will need when he is leaping. With my first baby, having never heard of the Wonder Weeks, I was slow to realise that a change was taking place during the first leap. I was baffled because what my baby had enjoyed up until that point suddenly seemed unsatisfactory. I had finally started to feel like I knew what I was doing, when suddenly I found myself completely at sea again, with no clue what was wrong, or what to do about it. My mother had to point out to me that my baby was bored and wanted me to talk to him. Believe it or not, that hadn't even occurred to me.

'A word of consolation: [a] demanding baby could be gifted. Some babies catch on to new games and toys quickly, soon growing tired of doing the same things, day in and day out. They want new challenges, continual action, complicated games and lots of variety. It can be extremely exhausting for mothers of these "bubbly" babies, because they run out of imagination, and their infants scream if they are not presented with one new challenge after another. It is a proven fact that many highly gifted children were demanding, discontented babies. They were usually happy only as long as they were offered new and exciting challenges.'[5]

The needs of a highly sociable, intelligent or extrovert baby can certainly be overwhelming for a new mother. It calls for energy, ingenuity and patience. It's as important to go to antenatal classes in order to build a social support network as it is to prepare for birth. Having a group of buddies with babies really comes into its own when he's becoming more socially alert, because it can be really hard work filling the days with enough interesting interactions to keep him content. I'll say it again: babies expect to be born into the Village when they arrive on this planet. By the end of the day, they are bored of seeing the same face, the same room and the same toys. They want new things to wrap their growing brains around. I had to take mine out every day, often several times a day, just to see people and the world outside, even if I had no specific place to go. Rainy days when the streets were empty and days when no one was free to meet up were especially tough. During a leap, the days often seemed like they would never end. My babies would fuss and cry and refuse to sleep, and I would rack my brains for ways to keep them happy. Before I had them I envisaged myself pottering around the house while they played happily with pots and pans, but that didn't happen. From the time my babies were just a few weeks old, I often got the distinct impression that they were wondering, *Where the hell is everyone?*

11) ROME WASN'T BUILT IN A DAY

'During the first 20 months of a baby's life, there are ten developmental leaps with their corresponding fussy periods at onset. The fussy periods come at 5, 8, 12, 15, 23, 34, 42, 51, 60 and 71 weeks. The onsets may vary by a week or two, but you can be sure of their arrival [...] The initial fussy phases your baby goes through as an infant do not last long. They can be as short as a few days – although they often seem longer to parents distressed over an infant's inexplicable crying [...] Later on the changes your infant undergoes become more complex, they take longer for her to assimilate and the fussy periods may last from 1 to 6 weeks.'[6]

The leaps are spaced just far enough apart that there is a brief window in between when babies seem a little more settled. But the drama of the next leap is never far away, and it all starts pretty early on. Around three to four weeks after birth, a baby's head circumference increases dramatically and the glucose metabolism in his brain changes.[7] The baby is gearing up for his first developmental leap since birth (the leaps are believed to begin in utero, but these have not been identified): 'Between four and five weeks old, your baby goes through a whole set of changes that affect his senses – the way he experiences the world, the way he feels, even the way he digests his food. His whole world feels, looks, smells and sounds different.'[8]

During this and every subsequent leap he will probably regress a little bit. He will be clingy and fretful and difficult to soothe. He probably won't want to sleep – or at least not alone – and he may be distant or go off his food. At these times it is easy to think that all our love and attention is spoiling him, or worry that he might be becoming 'difficult'. But very often the leaps end just as suddenly as they begin. For me, these anxieties returned with every new leap, and every time, my fears were unfounded. Once they came through the leap, my babies bounded forwards of their own accord and they seemed to take great pride and pleasure in doing so. A fussy phase or regression is not an indication that a baby needs sleep training or a stricter routine. Quite the opposite. A baby regresses because he needs extra help to get through his days and his nights. He needs to feel that you are a port in the storm – a safe place to cling to in the maelstrom of changing sensations.

As the weeks and months pass, babies experience one change after another. Van de Rijt and Plooij defined them as the 'worlds' of:

» **CHANGING SENSATIONS** (starting between 4.5 and 5 weeks) – a rapid maturation of metabolism, internal organs and senses
» **PATTERNS** (starting between 7.5 and 8.5 weeks) – becoming able to perceive patterns with all his senses outside and inside his body
» **SMOOTH TRANSITIONS** (starting between 11.5 and 12.5 weeks) – begins to move around in a less stiff or robotic way than before
» **EVENTS** (starting between 14.5 and 19.5 weeks) – becomes able to perceive a short series of smooth transitions such as grasping something with his hand
» **RELATIONSHIPS** (starting between 22.5 and 26.5 weeks) – a perception of the relationship between things: inside, outside, on top of, next to, underneath or in between – realises you can be far away from him!
» **CATEGORIES** (starting between 33.5 and 37.5 weeks) – perceiving similarities and differences and the ability to 'group' things accordingly
» **SEQUENCES** (starting between 41.5 and 46.5 weeks)

   – recognising and managing the flow of events and relationships over time, for example, eating with a spoon

» **PROGRAMS** (starting between 50.5 and 54.5 weeks) – understanding the idea behind putting a whole series of actions together in order to complete a task or produce a result, such as washing dishes or building a tower

» **PRINCIPLES** (starting between 59.5 and 64.5 weeks) – looking for boundaries; understanding the rules that govern the way things happen, especially with regards to social interactions

» **SYSTEMS** (starting between 70.5 and 76.5 weeks) – a toddler no longer applies principles as rigidly as before and is able to adjust according to circumstances: the earliest beginnings of a conscience

Each leap builds on the connections made and skills learnt during the previous one. They are sequential and though every baby masters different skills at different times, depending on his individual character, the mental building blocks are always laid down in the same order and at roughly the same age. If you know your baby's calculated due date, then you can work out when the storm is coming and the knowledge of this can turn the experience of a leap completely on its head – from stressful to wonderful. These are the Wonder Weeks.

'Even without an instruction manual, you know that your baby will explore each "new world" in his own individual way. You know that the best thing you can do is to "listen" to your baby, in order to help him on his way. You know how to have fun with him. You also know that you are the person who understands him best, and the person who can really help him unlike any other.'[9]

8. TOTALLY POTTY

The past is a foreign country: they do things differently there.
– L.P. Hartley

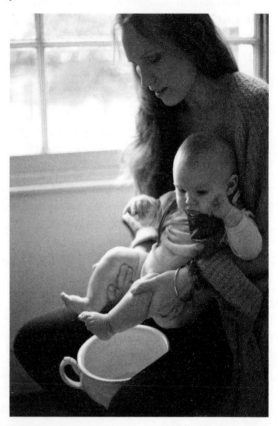

I) ALL GONE TO POT

'But aren't they like mice? Don't they just wee all the time?' were the words of my friend when I told her I was using a potty with my new baby. She was being polite but I suspect she was really thinking, *Are you mad? What the hell are you doing?* She's not alone in thinking that babies are incontinent and oblivious to their own bodily functions. It's what we are told by the experts and they're right to some extent. Babies who are put in nappies for the first two years of their lives do not develop the necessary awareness to participate in pottying. But babies who are offered the potty early on will learn to go on cue. I know because I have seen it for myself. Most childcare professionals are adamant that it is not physically possible for babies to control their bodies in this way and many say that to offer them the chance to learn 'too early' could even be damaging. As surely as night follows day, the need for nappies is written into our collective consciousness as a fact.

Nobody seems to even question the *fact* that, as a society, the more nappies we are using the longer our children seem to need them. You can buy 'pyjama pants' (nappies) for children aged 8 to 15 years old in supermarkets now. These are not aimed at children with special needs, but ordinary folk who still struggle with regular bed-wetting. Schools and nurseries are having to deal with children who are not fully toilet independent at later and later ages. And though teachers despair about having to deal with the consequences of this state of affairs in class, they too believe that there is a golden moment in a child's development when they will suddenly be ready to potty-train. A friend received a letter home from her child's nursery which explained to parents the correct way to potty-train their children. It stipulated that infants have *no control* over their sphincter muscles before they are 18 months old. And yet, by that same age (having introduced him to the potty at six months), I no longer needed to put nappies on my own son. He did not soil himself and was able to wait or 'hold on' until he or I suggested it was time to go to the loo. Was this a fluke? Is he a freak of nature? The answer is no.

A couple of generations ago, for a child to be clean and dry by 18 months would not have been unusual. Mothers would have held their babies over a potty and expected something to come out from around the age of six months, if not before.

There was no doubt in people's minds that a baby was able to actively pass waste, given the opportunity. The only real question was how soon would he be willing and able to hold on long enough to get to a potty by himself. In a household manual dating from 1878, mothers are advised: 'Children can be taught cleanliness, by putting a vessel under their lap when there is a sign of evacuation and will soon be not content to do without it. This practice may be begun at five or six weeks.'[1] People used nappies as a means to get on with life, because of how often babies needed to go, not because they thought they were incontinent. If you had to wash all those cloth nappies every day, you were rightly inclined to get the learning process underway as soon as possible. In the 1950s, 18 months was not considered an early age for potty-training.

It's not just that parents today are more forgiving of our children. Ironically, by denying our babies the chance to learn waste management early on, we saddle them with the harder task of unlearning what we set in place from the start. Encouraging babies to soil nappies means that this becomes normal and sometimes even preferable for them. But allowing them to poo in a reclined position is not conducive to a successful bowel movement and may prevent things moving through as well as they should. All in all, delaying potty-training until it can be done quickly and easily might actually make the process more fraught, costly and complicated than it needs to be. So how did we get here?

The big change came about in 1961 when Procter & Gamble (P&G) launched Pampers, a quick, clean alternative to washable nappies. At a time when many women were starting to look beyond the role of housewife for themselves, this revolutionary new product made combining a career and a family a bit easier. Super-absorbent gel was introduced in the 1980s, which meant babies could comfortably wear the same nappy for hours on end, reducing the work of constant changing. Disposables meant that we could spend money rather than time on our babies' nappies. It was an important part of the jigsaw that came together and enabled women to step out into a world of new opportunities. We ran with it, and for a while it all made perfect sense. But there are problems with disposable nappies that mean some people don't feel entirely comfortable using them any more. Modern washables are the answer for some, but for others there is another way.

Elimination communication (EC), infant potty-training (IPT), baby-led potty-training (BLPT) and natural infant hygiene (NIH) are all names that describe a relatively new movement based on a very old idea. I prefer to call it EC, because communication is the key element for me and I tend not to think of it as having much to do with traditional potty-training. In actual fact, we don't even use a potty most of the time, so it may be misleading to evoke the idea of a potty when we talk about it. More often than not I am holding my baby over something, be it a toilet, washing-up bowl, drain or grassy verge, because if you expect your baby to just sit on a potty and do his business then you're not going to get very far. Think of it as a collaborative effort – your body is a key element in helping him to know when to go.

Whatever you call it, the premise is that if you start early, you can harness a baby's inbuilt reflexes and instincts to gradually teach him to use a potty or go on cue when held. They still do it in India, in Africa, in China. In fact, it's being done right at this moment in places all over the world, so why do so many doctors say that it isn't possible? Because in the developed world it is commercially lucrative to convince parents not to. In 1962, Dr T. Berry Brazelton wrote about potty-training 'readiness' and this is still the benchmark paper on which much of the potty-training advice we are given is based. Brazelton wrote about the pitfalls of early potty-training, particularly at around 12 months when there is a developmental phase during which babies might become resistant and uncooperative about using a potty. This is typically the time when the early infantile reflexes have diminished but voluntary control has not yet been mastered. He reasoned that delaying potty-training until after 18 months would make the process quick and easy.

This was music to the ears of P&G, because it suggested that it was better to delay beginning any kind of potty-training until a whole year later than was considered normal at the time. They teamed up with Brazelton, funded his research and created the Pampers Parenting Institute, which went on to produce recommendations for later and later toilet training. They also produced a TV show for him to host and he featured in several Pampers commercials promoting the 'wait until they're ready' approach.[2] Once again, just as in the case of the infant formula industry, the potential to make a large profit meant that P&G were not content to simply meet an existing need. With a sprinkling of 'scientific' gold dust on top of their marketing campaigns, P&G convinced the public that nappies were not just convenient, but necessary. This is another in a long line of products whose sales figures benefit from the perpetration of the idea that human bodies don't work properly.

Brazelton was right that if you try to force a child to go to the loo in a way that he is unfamiliar or uncomfortable with, or that involves coercion, punishment or shame, you run the risk of causing him psychological harm. He was also correct in saying that there are times when your best efforts will be met with resistance from your child. The fussy phases of the Wonder Weeks are always interesting (see chapter 7). But this resistance is not a sign that the child is incapable and there are plenty of tricks to get around it. The nature of bringing up a child is that there are challenges along the way. The important thing is to let him know that you are with him. You move forward together as a team. You enable him to learn, you don't teach. With EC there is no rush, but ironically, children who do it are usually clean and dry earlier than those who don't.

Elimination communication should not be confused with conventional potty-training. In her book *Nappy Free Baby*,

Amber Hatch describes the three stages of development which your baby goes through as he learns to use a potty through EC. The first is the *reflex phase*, which is present at birth but fades by around four to six months. If you start pottying your baby before this reflex disappears, you can create a *conditioned response* (stage two) whereby the baby will open his sphincter on cue (most often a *shhhhh* sound). However, somewhere around 12 months the development of *voluntary control* (stage three) will interfere with the conditioned response: this is the grey period Brazelton referred to, when parents may become confused by their child's apparent regression. But this couple of months is only a blip in the grand scheme of things and for the baby it is an important shift towards autonomy. EC babies will soon return to pottying and go on to develop excellent control and awareness.

This is a long-term approach. There are no reward charts or do-it-in-a-week programmes. In one sense, EC is incredibly simple. You take your baby's nappy off when you think he might need the loo. If he goes, then great. If he doesn't, then you try again later. But not much later, because if one thing is guaranteed with babies, it's that there are *lots* of opportunities to catch something. From the day we start, we gradually develop a rhythm and a kind of communication that is hard to define and different for everyone. We start to know when he might need to go, just like we know when he's tired or hungry and even if we're not 100 per cent sure, it's just worth a try because elimination is as important a bodily function to respond to as any other. And like all the other skills he learns, it doesn't come overnight. Practice makes perfect, and the sooner we start the better.

11) NO-NAPPY HAPPY

Every new generation needs a revolution.
– Thomas Jefferson

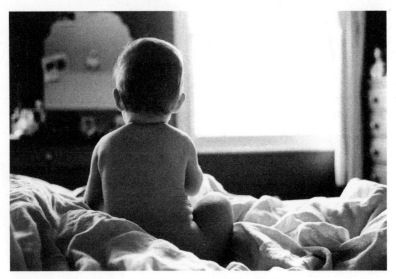

People are talking about EC and it is starting to gain momentum as a movement, but to read about it or hear about it from someone else is *not* how you discover EC. The moment you really discover EC is when you try it for yourself and there's nothing quite like your first time. It's when you take up your baby in a new way and hold him out in a squatting position. You might feel awkward and a bit apprehensive but when your baby instinctually responds, delivering a neat little deposit into a receptacle which can then be cleaned, it is one of those moments in life when the stars align and the universe suddenly makes sense. Eureka! So *that's* what people did before nappies were invented. It is a profound moment of connection with the wider world, human nature and our entire history. That's saying a lot for catching a poo in a pot, but that's honestly what it felt like to me. EC makes sense on so many levels, it's a shame that it's so marginal in our culture. There are lots of reasons why we could all benefit from a little more waste awareness in our lives:

» **BETTER OUT THAN IN.** Babies who can effectively release waste will be more comfortable and potentially less fretful.

» **LESS NAPPY RASH.** A little fresh air goes a long way. And let's face it, nobody should have to sit in a dirty nappy.

» **LESS CHANCE OF A BABY HOLDING ON OR GETTING CONSTIPATED.** The squatting position makes for regular and thorough 'evacuations'. No more poo-splosions up the back of his Babygro when he's little, and less chance of poos getting stuck inside him when he starts solids.

» **FEWER DIRTY NAPPIES TO CHANGE.** This means you either wash or buy less. Win-win.

» **A BABY LEARNS TO LISTEN TO HIS OWN BODY, AS WELL AS CONTROL IT.** This can only be a good thing.

» **PARENTS LEARN TO LISTEN TO THEIR BABY.** Feeling that you understand your baby is empowering.

» **A BABY LEARNS TO COMMUNICATE HIS NEEDS.** If your child grows up feeling that his needs are understood and considered valid you have given him a life-long gift.

» **REDUCED ENVIRONMENTAL IMPACT.** Western baby care weighs heavily on our carbon footprint (and on my personal parenting guilt-o-meter). I am grateful for anything that lightens the load.

» **ANYONE CAN DO EC.** Parents, grandparents, childminders, nannies, friends and neighbours. Whoever is looking after your baby, EC provides a genuine and rewarding bonding opportunity. It's certainly more fun than the 'bum job' of nappy duty.

» **EC BABIES USUALLY 'GRADUATE' AROUND THE AGE OF TWO.** This means you can get on with life and stop thinking about nappies.

There are also reasons why EC is a difficult choice to make, especially in our culture:

» **GETTING MESSY.** If you allow lots of nappy-free time, there is no doubt that you will sometimes get wee and poo on you, and possibly on your carpet. It all depends on how you feel about that. Baby poo can be a tough stain if you don't get it out straight away (ordinary soap and warm water works), but it doesn't really smell bad until you introduce solids. If you only offer the potty at nappy changes, there is little chance of any mess, but the communication aspect will be minimal, your baby might be less fussed about soiling nappies and you might feel less like the process is actually working. I found more baby clothes were ruined with my first son, *before* we started EC, because the nappies couldn't contain the three-day poo-splosions. There's no way around it, babies are just plain messy.

» **COLD CLIMATES.** Clothes can be a major obstacle to EC so a cold climate can be very frustrating. The poppers, the buttons, the onesies, and all those layers! But it can be done. Drop-flap nappies, leg warmers and split-crotch pants can all make life easier.

» **OUT AND ABOUT.** Unless you are having a nice walk in the countryside, ECing while out and about can be tricky, because with EC, when nature calls, you have to answer, even if there is no baby-change facility nearby. With an older baby, he might be able to hold on for a few minutes, but little ones have to go when they have to go. In a drain, behind a tree, on the hard shoulder of the motorway. I can't count the number of times I have undressed a baby on my knee in a public loo, trying not to let any part of me or him touch anything unpleasant. At moments like that, I sometimes wonder why I bother. The main problem is our culture is not set up for EC. But the more people who do it the more likely it is that this will change.

» **FEELING LIKE A FREAK.** This really depends on the individual. Some people practising EC will have lots of friends who also do it. Some won't know anyone else at all. It can be challenging if you have little or no support.

I fell into EC through necessity, but as is so often the case in life, a bad situation ended up revealing a new path. You might have to see it to believe it, but once you start to believe in EC, there's no going back.

When our first baby was six months old, we finally plucked up the gusto to go on holiday (I say holiday, we managed to travel 130 miles to the coast). We had recently started him on solids, and everyone was encouraging me to feed him up, because he was quite big and the general consensus seemed to be that milk would not be enough for him any more. People said that he would fuss less and sleep better once he felt 'properly' full. Unfortunately he just became hopelessly constipated and more unsettled than ever. I knew about 'baby-led weaning', but I thought that was more to do with avoiding fussy eating habits, and my health visitor had advised me to offer a combination of purees and finger foods. I failed to make the connection between the stubborn poo and the solid food and I worked hard to chop, cook, blend, divide up and freeze enough vegetable goop in advance to last us for the whole holiday.

A couple of days into the trip we went out for a long walk. With him in the sling, it felt good to stretch our legs and we were looking forward to a great view at the top of a steep cliff. He was fussing as usual, and I was trying to distract him with songs, jiggling and occasionally trying to feed him. He hadn't pooped for a week, but that wasn't unusual for him. After an hour or so he started getting really upset. He was wriggling, straining and grunting. When we reached a break in the trees at one of the outlook points, I untied the sling and set him down on a bench. I stripped off his nappy and he finally let his poo go, whilst literally kicking and screaming. It was enormous and hard and I know it really hurt him. That day is etched in my memory and shall forever be known in our family as 'the poo with a view'. What should have been a lovely day became an absolute misery because I had no idea how to listen or connect to my baby about his elimination needs.

I will always regret that experience, but nevertheless it was a turning point. After that, both my mum and mother-in-law suggested we try him on a potty to see if that could help get things moving. We bought one, but I wasn't sure what to do with it. One day I was reading about parenting in other cultures in *The Other Baby Book* while he was asleep on my lap. The book described the basic principles of EC. It was the first I had ever heard of it, but once I had read those pages it was as if I had always known about it. It was just so glaringly obvious. Of course people in places without nappies don't spend the whole day soaked in excrement! Of course there is a simple solution. It gave me the nudge I needed to try the potty. When he woke up I whisked him to the bathroom and sat him on the potty, half expecting nothing at all. But to my utter amazement he did a wee and a poo right there and then as if it was no big thing. There was really no turning back after that. Just giving it a go was the key to finding a thrilling new way to connect with my baby. I felt I had discovered an untapped portal into his wordless little world. How often had he cried and I had been baffled? How many times had he tried to tell me? I felt robbed, suddenly aware of all the missed opportunities there had been over the past six months. But at the same time, what a gift! From now on I would be listening.

The communication aspect of EC is not just between parent and baby. It's also about allowing a baby's body to develop a clear line of communication within itself. The act of urinating is dictated by two sets of sphincter. The internal sphincter responds to a full bladder and this message is managed by the spinal cord, making this an *involuntary* feedback response. But in order for the urine to be released it must pass through another ring of muscle. The external sphincter is the gatekeeper and it is controlled by the conscious brain. This is a *voluntary* response which the baby or child will eventually learn to control. But this response is highly subject to conditioning.

> 'From birth, but most noticeably in the two-to-ten-month period, the sphincter becomes *conditioned* to release in set circumstances. After a few weeks (or even days) of holding your baby out and catching his urine, your baby begins to make an association between the hold, or perhaps the sound, or the feel of the pot on his buttocks (or a combination of these things), and the action of passing urine. This creates a *conditioned response* [...] Conditioning takes place whether you desire it or not. When babies use nappies conventionally, their infantile reflexes fade after a couple of months, to be replaced by a conditioned response to urinate and defecate in their nappies (sometimes waiting until a fresh nappy is put on before urinating).'[3]

The bowel works in a similar way, with two sets of sphincter, the external of which being under voluntary control (though in a young baby this is not 'conscious' control in the way we think of it in older children and adults). In the first few weeks and months, babies are very affected by their own bodies. They are experiencing the sensations of food passing through them and the resultant discomfort for the first time. This means that they will often signal strongly when they need to wee or poo. But we are generally not looking for these signs, and as time passes, babies become more accustomed to these feelings and they also become more interested in events outside their own bodies. This early signalling phase therefore usually passes without us having taken advantage of it.[4] When we encourage babies to pass waste into a nappy, we engineer the need to retrain their bodies later on, in order to rebuild the lost connection. In times past, the discomfort of a wet or dirty nappy would have made it harder for babies to ignore what was going on down there, but modern nappies don't even feel wet, so many babies would be happy to use them indefinitely.

Unfortunately, nappy use is much like any other consumer habit. Once you start, and once it becomes an accepted part of the culture, it's hard to stop. Like caffeine, alcohol and sugar, our culture is hooked on nappies; dependent and oblivious (or in denial) about their ill effects. Countries that remain largely untroubled by such a dependency pose a challenge for manufacturers like Procter & Gamble, who have been trying to establish a taste for nappies in China for many, many years.

'Western consumer goods companies take a proven product from overseas and introduce it in an emerging market with no prior knowledge of the products' use or existence [...] taking a product and literally changing consumer behavior to create a market for it [...] P&G had a terrible time launching Pampers in China, because Chinese consumers simply did not see a need for disposable diapers. Between traditional cloth diapers and *kaidangku*, Chinese mothers felt that they had their babies covered. After P&G did some research to identify the winning qualities of a disposable diaper in China, they put their marketing machine to work: Pampers launched the "Golden Sleep" campaign in 2007, which included mass carnivals and in-store campaigns in China's biggest urban areas [...] The ad campaign boasted "scientific" results, such as "Baby Sleeps with 50% Less Disruption" and "Baby Falls Asleep 30% Faster." Pampers now ranks No. 1 in a product category that barely existed just a few years ago.'[5]

These *kaidangku* pants are the key to the traditional Chinese approach. And they work a treat. 'Chinese parents have their children potty trained to some degree before the age of eighteen months, if not much sooner.'[6] They don't have a particular name for the practice because it is a routine part of baby care, and has been for as long as anyone can remember. 'Around three months or a hundred days, when the baby has more head and neck control, he is held over a basin when he has to go [...] An entire household and even community share in the responsibility of training.'[7] In India too, the culture is totally geared towards early infant waste awareness. As Laurie Boucke explains:

'Extended families are still commonplace in villages, so a mother has plenty of help from other women and girls in the household [...] Babies spend most of their time in-arms, either sitting on their mother's lap or being carried by her or one of the other women in the home [...] The baby usually sleeps on the mother's chest or right next to her, without diapers. A mother is so attuned to her baby that she automatically wakes up during the night when it is time for her baby to go.'[8]

Though EC is more widely used in the UK than you might think, it is still undoubtedly an unusual parenting choice. And the fact that it is a *choice*, rather than commonplace, as it is in China, makes it challenging. As Amber Hatch, the author of *Nappy Free Baby*, points out, 'The choices available to parents today can allow us to make enlightened decisions about the way we raise our babies. They can also leave us feeling bewildered and unsupported, especially if we go against the grain of popular culture.'[9] Imagine living in a culture where everyone adopted similar parenting techniques. Imagine not feeling confused, defensive and exhausted by our choices all the time. Imagine being able to ask for advice from our friends and being certain that they knew exactly what we were talking about. Imagine if our parents understood and supported us unconditionally in what we were doing, and even knew how to help without instruction.

'In countries where early potty training is the norm, mothers can ask any woman for advice; everyone understands the merits of helping their baby to void in an appropriate place. Also, mothers are simply expected to start potty training from birth, so there is no conscious decision to be made – they aren't going against convention. This makes practicing the method so much easier – especially in the early days.'[10]

There's no doubt that EC is harder to do if you don't know anyone else doing it. It can add to the loneliness of parenting, but it can also be a channel for finding kindred spirits. As with breastfeeding, EC can be a daunting prospect if you have no prior or first-hand experience of it. It's a good idea to seek out other people who are doing it and to witness it in action. You will find that different people do it in different ways, depending on their circumstances, their motivations and their baby's preferences. There are also books that describe the process in detail with lots of information to get you started and help you through the challenges you encounter. You might find that members of previous generations remember early potty-training from when they were young, and can provide some help and advice. And as always, the online community of people practising EC are an invaluable resource for information, encouragement and EC-friendly clothing. Here Hatch points out all the reasons she and so many of us genuinely enjoy EC:

'[M]any parents who help their baby pass waste don't even consider themselves to be potty training. For them, the benefits of offering the potty are entirely self-evident, in the moment. *They enjoy the process for its own sake.* They know how to help their baby pass a difficult stool; they can soothe and settle their baby at night; they enjoy his delight as he wees on the bushes. They love the confidence it gives them in handling their baby and communicating with him. They enjoy saving nappies. They enjoy knowing why he may be unsettled. This experience teaches us that potty training doesn't have to be "a necessary evil" – to be crammed into as short a time as possible.'[11]

III) THE ROAD LESS TRAVELLED: EC FROM BIRTH

When my second son was born, he was held over a potty from day one and I kept a diary of the experience.

WEEK 1 – Day one and we have a whole poo and half a wee catch. I can't believe it. I'm in a daze after the birth and not focused on EC at all, so Luke is the one who gives it a go. He feels like a superhero!

WEEK 2 – Lots of catches, but it doesn't seem to just be down to timing or coincidence. He really responds to being 'held out', especially at night. And it genuinely feels like communication – it's probably the only kind of communication we have right now.

WEEK 3 – I use cloth for two nights in a row and he gets nappy rash. He is really unsettled and has started crying a lot. It seems like madness to add EC to an already full plate. I'm wondering why we are doing this to ourselves, and I resolve to ease off a bit.

WEEK 4 – Despite my doubts, it seems like EC is part of the solution to the crying, so we persevere. Sometimes I think he waits to have his nappy taken off, and often gets cross when he needs to go. Is it possible that he already expects this? One night I only use two nappies because he wakes and I catch – but that means not much sleep for me. I can't decide if this is fantastic or awful.

WEEK 5 – Starting to develop a rhythm. After a feed I offer the potty and usually get a wee, sometimes a poo. Then I keep the nappy off and put a washable pad under his bum while I'm holding him because 10 minutes later he gets fussy and

MY EC PHRASEBOOK

POTTITUNITY: Anytime, anywhere. When nature calls, we answer.

CATCH: An opportunity to bask in parenting glory for about three minutes, until the baby pukes on me or I walk past a mirror and realise I have porridge in my hair.

MISS: An opportunity to practise my Zen-like ability to 'let go of the goal'. Mop up and move on.

NEAR MISS: I knew it! I totally knew it, but I either second-guessed myself, or I just wasn't quick enough. Better luck next time.

POONAMI: This is a code-red situation where all available hands must scramble to help deal with the deluge. It's the poo that just keeps on coming!

THE ONE-HANDED-WET-WIPE-WIGGLE: Getting those blighters out of the packet with one hand is an important skill and essential when single-handedly holding the baby over the potty and dealing with a poonami. When you EC from birth, be prepared to learn to juggle!

THE ONE-HANDED-TOILET-TISSUE-TEAR: A similar problem but a different technique. Holding the baby on one arm and trying to liberate a sheet from the roll is about as tricky as it gets, but with patience anyone can master the art.

if I offer, it's another wee. This can go on until I put a nappy back on for the next nap.

WEEK 6 – Three poo catches in one day, one of which was in a friend's bathroom sink. She was okay with it.

WEEK 7 – Six weeks brings the first smiles but with it some almighty evening screaming sessions. Sadly the 'witching hour' is considerably longer than an hour. We've been using Gaviscon on and off because the midwife thinks he's fussy due to reflux, but it doesn't seem to make any difference and I'm in two minds about the whole thing. It definitely makes his poo thicker, and I worry it's blocking him up.

He seems to prefer to poo at night. One night he poos at every waking – that's five times!

WEEK 8 – A quick trip to the shops takes longer than I expect and although I have a spare nappy with me, I have nothing else – I have NO WET WIPES! I feed bub in a cafe and take him to the loo where he does an enormous poo straight into the toilet. I wipe and dress him without any mess or fuss. A moment of glory.

WEEK 9 – Wonder Week chaos begins. General brain-growth grumpiness means quite a lot of indignant refusals and subsequent misses.

I catch a poo in my next-door neighbour's loo and feel somehow relieved. I realise I feel a self-imposed pressure to perform when around non-ECers, lest I 'fail' publicly and am judged a complete loony.

A night with one dry nappy for the whole 12 hours. Every wake-up we caught the wee. Amazing.

WEEK 10 – Immunisations bring fever, screaming, a night of full nappies and general misery.

We run out of disposables so I brave the cloth again. We use drop-flap nappies (Flaparaps are our favourite) which make EC much easier, as they are so quick and easy to open and close. We do really well with them at night, but I find he does too many little wees in the daytime and it makes a lot of extra washing. I plan to buy more disposables but somehow manage to unselect them when checking out my online shopping, so they don't arrive with the rest of the delivery. It must have been an unconscious decision to keep going with cloth.

Only one or two poos a day now. On one hand this is great, but I do spend the whole time on high alert, anticipating a poo that never comes.

WEEK 11 – I start using a washing-up bowl at night-time. Why didn't I think of that before? You literally can't miss!

WEEK 12 – The nappy rash comes back so I buy some disposables. I have a real love / hate relationship with cloth.

WEEK 14 – Wonder Week over. Consistent catching recommences. What a relief!

WEEK 15 – I have tonsillitis and have to take antibiotics, which gives him the runs. One night we get through seven nappies!

WEEK 17 – My 11-day course of antibiotics is finally over and I'm ecstatically happy to see regular poos return. I breathe a sigh of relief but before the week is out we spend a night in hospital because he has a chest infection. He has to start his own course of antibiotics and within hours he has the runs again – green and bitty and totally unpredictable. I make it through the night ECing with an absorbent mat. The nurses are a bit baffled.

I give him probiotics and it makes his poo smell like Yakult.

WEEK 18 – I feel despondent and defeated by difficult circumstances. We were making good progress in the first couple of months but after relying on nappies during all the tummy trouble I feel he has lost the inclination to communicate about things a little bit. Maybe it's just part of the regression during leap four (this is a long leap).

WEEK 19 – He has started letting me know when he needs to go again and at night the nappies are virtually always dry when he stirs for a wee. I don't know whether it is a coincidence, but he's entering the second stage of leap four this week and he does suddenly seem much more in control of himself. People have been remarking that he looks more mature all of a sudden, as if he has his wits about him.

WEEK 20 – Pop-up tissues! The answer! Why didn't I think of it sooner? You don't really need a wet wipe unless the poo is dried on and smeared around (which it never is when you use a potty). I've been wiping with wet wipes and then drying his bum before putting the nappy back on. (I know!!) What an absolute game-changer. Tissues are cheaper, more eco and can be flushed. I'm genuinely excited about pop-up tissues.

WEEK 21 – He poos in threes. After I wipe he goes again. Usually there are three instalments, the last of which is a bubbly fizz!

WEEK 23 – It's hard to measure any 'progress' because it's all so gradual. But it's lovely to see EC develop alongside all the other clever things he's learning. This process takes time, but we're not in any hurry.

WEEK 24 – Having felt all calm and collected about things last week, I'm now losing the will to live. I cannot be sick and look after sick children ANY MORE! Ten weeks of non-stop illness means I am run into the ground and totally relying on disposables. I look at the cloth nappies sitting there, waiting to be put to use and feel a pang of failure. I think if I didn't have a three-year-old to look after, or I had anyone else around to help me with EC, we would be doing a bit better. (After a strong start, Luke has completely thrown in the towel.) But it's Christmas soon, so let's have some sherry and cheer up! On the plus side, we only use a couple of nappies a day, they're never full and he definitely knows what he's doing; he will try for me even if I've just missed it (which I usually have).

WEEK 25 – Five months old! Bub can sit on a potty now. I feel ridiculously proud and he's so chuffed with himself. He grins and I think he knows he's clever. Amazing that such sweet moments can come from catching poo!

WEEK 26 – Christmas Day with the in-laws. We make catches all day long to rounds of applause and praise for the 'clever' baby. He is clever, as all babies are, but I feel grumpy that my part in this whole potty process is overlooked. Am I being oversensitive? I'm not sure.

WEEK 27 – He falls asleep on my lap with no nappy on, which is not planned, but not a complete disaster either. After 20 minutes he starts to stir, fusses for a moment, wees (into the folded muslin I have strategically placed there to catch it), then goes back to sleep. Did he stir because he needed a wee, or did he wee because he stirred? I ponder the age-old question of night-time dryness. Lots of people say their babies/toddlers/children wee in their sleep. But I think it's not that simple. There is a pattern to it and as they get older, they can last for longer, but they do stir for a wee, whether they wake up or not.

WEEK 29 – I can put him in split-crotch pants for a couple of hours and catch everything now. I just can't bake a cake with my three-year-old while he's wearing them. Then there will be poo on the floor.

WEEK 30 – Six months! How strange to be here, at the age when we started EC with my first. And how different the experience with our second has been. It's not that he is so much better at signalling or waiting for the potty. I just know that he knows that I know when he needs to go. And that is really very special. It's a connection at the end of the day and there is trust in there somewhere, so I am proud and thankful. And I love the fact that he poos every day, with no stress or build up. That feels healthy.

WEEK 35 – Seven months. I can see why lots of cultures around the world typically start this at six months. There has been a massive shift over the past couple of weeks. He is *really* getting it now. I can hardly believe it, but we haven't used nappies for a couple of weeks. NO NAPPIES! Not cloth, not disposables, not training pants. Just bare bum in trousers. DAY AND NIGHT. I'm not saying we won't have to start using them again when he has his next leap or cuts his first teeth. But this is really amazing.

WEEK 41 – Eight months. He has mastered crawling and one of the first things he did was to scramble over to a potty when he needed to go! At first I wasn't sure, but when he did it three times in one day, I realised what was going on. We haven't managed to learn the chest slap sign yet, but I guess this is as sure a sign as any. The effort is really starting to pay off now. What a marvellous adventure.

WEEK 46 – Nine months. He has two teeth and we haven't needed nappies for a couple of months now – day or night! I'm still pinching myself that this is even possible. He doesn't poo at night any more and sleeps through from eight till seven, waking to wee and feed every three hours or so. I feel fine and get enough sleep. And he really has control of himself when he goes. If he has a little accident, he usually just does a little bit and waits for me to whisk him to the potty where he does the rest. Amazing.

IV) EC-PEASY: TIPS TO GET YOU STARTED

Feel the fear and do it anyway.
– Susan Jeffers

There is no 'right' way to do EC because everyone's different and discovering your own tricks of the trade is part of the fun, but here are some tips that might make starting feel less bewildering.

WHEN?

As often as you can without letting it completely take over your life. EC is definitely more hassle in cold climates, so don't drive yourself to distraction with getting clothes on and off. Even once a day is better than never, and you may be surprised and glad to know that a baby will still get the idea even if it's only a part-time thing.

» **AFTER NAPS** – Babies tend to wee as soon as they wake up. If you're quick, you can catch it.

» **DURING OR AFTER A FEED** – Eating stimulates the bowel and if a baby is popping on and off the breast during a feed it could be that he's wrestling with the urge to go.

» **NAPPY-CHANGE TIME** – When the nappy comes off, you might find that your baby instinctively does a wee anyway. This is a natural reflex. Why not hold him over a potty for a minute; you might find you get a poo as well.

» **AT NIGHT** – When babies stir at night it isn't necessarily hunger that disturbs them. Try him over a bowl and if he goes, he may then settle better.

» **BABY CUES** – Many babies fuss or cry out when they need to go. It's worth trying, but you'll have to be quick or you'll miss it! If you use a sign for potty (usually putting your hand up to your chest), a baby can learn how to let you know long before he can talk.

» **ADULT CUES** – You can make a *shhhhhh* sound whenever the baby goes, to build an association. Very soon, making this sound will cue him to go 'on command'.

» **TIMING** – You might get to know your baby's patterns and be able to anticipate things.

» **INTUITION** – Some people develop something of a sixth sense about it. But if you don't, then don't beat yourself up about it; it doesn't mean you're not 'in tune' with your baby, it just means he will be a great poker player when he grows up! Seriously, don't sweat it.

» **WHEN YOU GO** – if you're already going to the loo, then why not?

WHERE?

Well, anywhere and everywhere really. It depends how bold you are. EC is not potty-training, and a potty is just one of a myriad of options open to you.

» **OUTDOORS** – Whether it's the fresh air around the nether regions or the distraction of the birds, the trees or the traffic, most babies seem to relax instantly when you take them outside. If you think he needs to go, but he is protesting for whatever reason, then just pop outdoors. This *always* works for us.

» **WASHING-UP BOWL** – When holding a small baby, it's really hard to anticipate where things are going to go, and wees and poos often fire in different directions. You can find attractive vintage chamber pots to dip the baby's whole bottom into, or I found a large enamel washing-up bowl was great for ensuring a mess was avoided.

» **SINK/BATH/TOILET** – Wherever you are around the house, you can potty your baby, and if there's a tap you can turn on, so much the better. I found running water often inspired my babies to go. Plus, the clean-up is a total breeze.

WHAT?

The great thing about EC is that once you get the hang of it, your change bag becomes virtually obsolete. You can streamline down to a couple of spare nappies or washable pads and some tissues. However, there are a few items of kit that do make life easier.

» **LEG WARMERS** – Great for giving you access to your little one's bottom without the rigmarole of taking clothes off. Baby will be happier about being pottied if it's quick, hassle-free and doesn't involve getting cold. You can buy them, but they're not cheap and tend to be a bit tight on chunky thighs. If you (or someone you know) can knit, make some out of real wool as it repels water. I just cut the feet off some long socks. They worked a treat.

» **DROP-FLAP NAPPIES** – These are a total game-changer, especially if you team them with leg warmers. No poppers or Velcro. No need to lay your baby on his back for a change. Go to bornready.uk to find out more about them.

» **TUPPERWARE** – You can buy a porta-potty with disposable bags that go underneath for when you're out and about, but a Tupperware box works well for younger babies that can't sit on a potty. Tupperware is cheap and comes in all shapes and sizes, so you can choose what works for you. Seal it up and then just wash it out whenever you can. Putting a tissue in the bottom of the tub in advance makes cleaning out a poo even easier.

» **POP-UP TISSUES** – By all means use washable wipes (cut squares of jersey or towelling fabric to make your own), but I found that having a tissue box in every room meant I could always wipe quickly and easily without scrabbling around for a wet wipe.

HOW?

» **HOLDING A BABY OUT** – When a baby is very young, you'll need to support his whole body along one forearm, against your body and clasp his thighs with your hands. Once he can hold his head up, you can support him in a sitting position, with his back against your tummy. Even if he is able to sit on a potty, this is not always the best option because babies sometimes lose interest in this and it gives him the option to resist – he can get up and crawl away! But if you hold him, there is a connection there which helps sometimes. You can hold him in front of a mirror and talk to him, or let him tinkle over some bushes outside. There are a lot of options open to you when you hold your baby out. Plus you get really strong!

WHO?

» **EVERYONE** – Encourage partners, grandparents, aunts and uncles, friends and neighbours to have a go. Once they get a catch, or feel that the baby is trying for them, they will be so much more enthusiastic about the idea. The temptation can be to do it on the sly when no one is looking. But it is so much easier when you have support, so don't be shy about it. Spread the word!

V) SEW SOME SPLIT-CROTCH PANTS

You can make your own split-crotch pants. You'll need half a metre of fabric and some elastic. You don't need a sewing machine. I like to use 100 per cent cotton jersey, just like my wrap slings. It's comfy, breathable and you don't have to hem it because it won't fray. There are sewing patterns available for free online. I added the flaps front and back to save my neighbours' blushes!

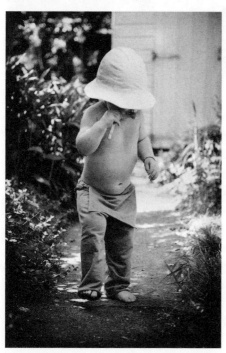

9. LOVE IS THE LAW

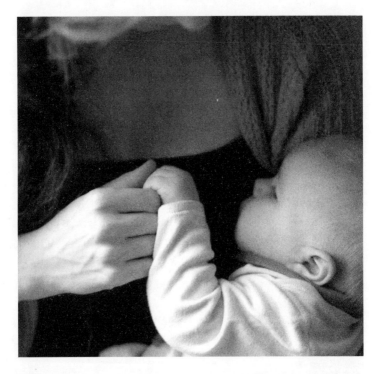

In *The Continuum Concept*, Jean Liedloff talks about how we have lost touch with what is truly 'right' for the way our species evolved to live.[1] As she explains, the human body is built with a set of expectations about the world it will emerge into. Ultimately the environment determines the form of every animal on earth, because we are each a product of every ancestor that has gone before us, and the survival of our genes has depended upon them being correct or advantageous for the habitat in which we live. A fish expects to emerge into water when he arrives on the planet and everything about him is built to suit that environment. Just as his gills and fins are an expectation of water, our human lungs are an expectation of air and our eyes are an expectation of light. In this way, everything about a baby can be said to have the expectation of a certain set of environmental conditions. These include near constant closeness to a primary caregiver, being fed without question when he is hungry, and being carried in arms until he is no longer helpless. The infants of our species evolved in these conditions, and this has enabled us to become what we are today. Like a joey in a pouch, the immediate environment a human baby expects and needs to become part of upon his emergence from the womb is the body of his mother, because he cannot survive without it. To remove him from his adaptive environment is like taking a fish out of water. He will flap and flail and buck his body, desperate to be returned to his right place.

Every baby's needs and preferences are unique, but his expectations are built into his DNA and they are legitimate, whatever they may be, no matter what society dictates. He asks only for what he needs in order to feel right and whole and human. Listen to your baby's needs and believe in them. Don't let anyone tell you they know better than you. No one knows your baby better than you do, because your baby *is* you. He is *made of you* and *you made him*. And you continue to make him every day after birth, so even if you are a non-biological parent, when you nurture your child, you build yourself into him, which makes him feel full and strong and assured. You are entering into a life-long commitment and as with any relationship, attempting to change a person as soon as you meet them will kill your relationship before it has come alive. Your baby is no exception. We are what we are and the first step is acceptance and understanding. You can help a person grow into the best version of themselves once you have established a bond of trust, but it is important that every baby grows up with the feeling that he is right and good just the way he is.

A baby is not a project to complete with top marks. 'Success' is not about getting your babies to sleep through the night, your children to finish what's on their plate or your teenagers to ace their exams. If anything, success is the weird and beautiful mess that can be found in the cracks between 'getting it right', meeting 'milestones' and following 'The Rules'. Getting it wrong is just as important, because that's when we are at our most raw and honest and human. That's when we learn something about ourselves. That's when the lacquer of perfection is stripped away and the rough surface underneath is revealed – a surface that can bond. The best feelings in life come from simple moments of pure connection, clarity and love. Beyond that, what else matters anyway?

Try not to look outwards for the answers – you have them within you. Accepting that there is no 'right' way of doing things will be the hardest thing I ever manage to do, if I ever manage it. But I know in my heart that the only right way is the way that works – for *my* family. It's the way that feels right, even if it goes against all the advice I am given. It's scary to defy convention, friends and relatives. But if you stand your ground and project only love, then people generally don't mind as much as you think they will. When they see that your baby is happy, most people will leave you be. They may even congratulate you.

As for the words of all the 'experts', remember that some of the greatest minds in medicine thought that babies couldn't feel pain 60 years ago. It is easy to become driven by the idea that there is an ultimate 'truth' or 'fact' or 'right' or 'wrong' to be found. But so often it all depends on how you look at it, where you are coming from and what you want to see. Our children depend on us to hold the answers, to decode the world and to reveal the truth. Mastering the ability to sort the wheat from the chaff is a rite of passage which distinguishes an adult from a child. We must all learn to hone our instincts if we are to see clearly what must be seen, what must be known, in order to make 'right' decisions. In this book, I have given examples of scientific findings which I believe to be correct. This is based on research, observation and ultimately my own instinct. But 'truth' is not a matter of absolutes. Evidence and advice change all the time, so don't take it too much to heart. If it feels right and good to you then it probably is. Enjoy your babies. They grow up fast.

ACKNOWLEDGEMENTS

Thank you, Shasta, for the beef stroganoff and the knitted booties, for *The Wonder Weeks* and the wise words.

You were a port in the storm.

You made it fun.

Thank you, Roz, for the softest crochet lemon-yellow blanket, for the fruit basket and the flowers.

You are my dearest friend.

Thank you, Luke, Mo, Carole, Brian and Mum.

You were my village.

You held things together when I could not.

Thank you, Carmen Pagor, Pauline Cross, Becky Reed, Jenn Philpott, Amber Hatch, Anna Lee, Hazel Jones and Natalie Hickman.

You inspired me.

Thank you, Martin, Maria, Zoë, Emma and Zoë.

You believed in me.

REFERENCES

2. A PREGNANT PAUSE

[1] Hopgood, *How Eskimos Keep Their Babies Warm*, p.152.

[2] Monbiot, 'Rewilding Our Children', *Guardian*, 17 April 2012.

[3] Paul, 'Radiant Zinc Fireworks Reveal Quality of Human Egg', *northwestern.edu*, 26 April 2016.

[4] Enright, *Making Babies*, p.3.

[5] Lokugamage, *The Heart in the Womb*, p.7.

[6] Lokugamage, *The Heart in the Womb*, p.64.

3. BELIEVING IN BIRTH

[1] Witman and Wall, 'The Evolutionary Origins of Obstructed Labor: Bipedalism, encephalization, and the human obstetric dilemma', *Obstetrical and Gynecological Survey* 62.11, 2007, p.740.

[2] Hodge in Gaskin, *Birth Matters*, p.59.

[3] dir. Harman and Wakeford, *Freedom for Birth*, 2012.

[4] *improvingbirth.org*, 2016.

[5] Wertz and Wertz, *Lying-in: A History of Childbirth in America*, p.122.

[6] Gaskin, *Birth Matter*, p.66.

[7] Gaskin, *Ina May's Guide to Childbirth*, p.246.

[8] Meenan et al., 'A New (Old) Manoeuvre for the Management of Shoulder Dystocia', *The Journal of Family Practice*, 1991, p.32.

[9] The World Health Organization: European Regional Office, 'Having a Baby in Europe', European Regional Office, 1985.

[10] Moorhead, 'Different Planets', *Guardian*, 3 Oct 2006.

[11] UNICEF, *The State of the World's Children*, 2008.

[12] OECD Health Data 2007; NCHS, 2008; Deaths, Final Data, 2005.

[13] Halfdansdottir et al., 'Outcome of Planned Home and Hospital Births among Low-Risk Women in Iceland in 2005–2009: A retrospective cohort study', *Birth* 42.1, 2015.

[14] Li et al., 'Perinatal and Maternal Outcomes in Planned Home and Obstetric Unit Births in Women at "Higher Risk" of Complications: Secondary analysis of the birthplace national prospective cohort study', *British Journal of Obstetrics and Gynaecology*, April 2015.

[15] Li et al., 'Perinatal and Maternal Outcomes in Planned Home and Obstetric Unit Births in Women at "Higher Risk" of Complications: Secondary analysis of the birthplace national prospective cohort study', *British Journal of Obstetrics and Gynaecology*, April 2015.

[16] dir. Pascale-Bonaro, *Orgasmic Birth*, 2009.

[17] Jones in dir. Pascale-Bonaro, *Orgasmic Birth*, 2009.

[18] Gaskin, *Birth Matters*, p.56.

[19] Gaskin, *Birth Matters*, p.32.

[20] Wagner in dir. Pascale-Bonaro, *Orgasmic Birth*, 2009.

[21] Sharkey et al., 'Melatonin Synergizes with Oxytocin to Enhance Contractility of Human Myometrial Smooth Muscle Cells', *The Journal of Clinical Endocrinology and Metabolism*, 2009.

[22] Lothian, 'Do Not Disturb: The Importance of Privacy in Labor', *The Journal of Perinatal Education*, 2004, p.4.

[23] Buckley in dir. Pascale-Bonaro, *Orgasmic Birth*, 2009.

[24] Gaskin in dir. Pascale-Bonaro, *Orgasmic Birth*, 2009.

[25] Aldrich et al., 'The Effect of Maternal Pushing on Fetal Cerebral Oxygenation and Blood Volume during the Second Stage of Labour', *British Journal of Obstetrics and Gynaecology* 102.6, June.

[26] Roberts et al., 'Second Stage Pushing: A comparison of Valsalva-style with "mini" pushing', *The Journal of Perinatal Education* 4.4, December 1995.

[27] Sampselle et al., 'Spontaneous Pushing During Birth: Relationship to perineal outcomes', *Journal of Midwifery and Women's Health* 44.1, January–February 1999.

[28] Littlejohn, *spiritualbirth.net*, 2014.

[29] Littlejohn, *spiritualbirth.net*, 2014

[30] Reed, 'The Anterior Cervical Lip: How to ruin a perfectly good birth', *Midwife Thinking*, 2015.

[31] Reed, 'The Anterior Cervical Lip: How to ruin a perfectly good birth', *Midwife Thinking*, 2015.

[32] Odent, 'Fetus Ejection Reflex and the Art of Midwifery', *wombecology.com*, 2016.

[33] Odent, 'Champagne and the Fetus Ejection Reflex', *Midwifery Today* 65, Spring 2003.

[34] Lu Gao et al., 'Steroid Receptor Coactivators 1 and 2 Mediate

Fetal-to-Maternal Signaling that Initiates Parturition', *Journal of Clinical Investigation* 125.7, June 2015.

[35] 'You and Your Baby at 37–40 Weeks Pregnant', *nhs.uk*, 2016.

[36] 'Ob-Gyns Redefine Meaning of "Term-Pregnancy"', *acog.org*, 2016.

[37] Smith, 2001 and Jukic et al., 2013 in Dekker, 'Evidence on Inducing Labor for Going Past Your Due Date', *evidencebasedbirth. com*, 2015.

[38] Rosenstein et al., 'Risk of Stillbirth and Infant Death Stratified by Gestational Age', *Obstetrics & Gynecology* 120.1, July.

[39] NICE Guidelines, 2008.

[40] Kendall-Tackett, Cong and Hale, 'Birth Interventions Related to Lower Rates of Exclusive Breastfeeding and Increased Risk of Postpartum Depression in a Large Sample', *Clinical Lactation* 6.3, 2015, p.87.

[41] King's College Hospital, 'Inner City Midwifery Care: New study results', *www.kcl.ac.uk*, 3 Oct 2001.

[42] 'Statistical Outcomes 1999–2007', *thealbanymodel.com*, 2015.

[43] Sandall et al., 'Midwife-led Continuity Models versus Other Models of Care for Childbearing Women', *Cochrane*, April 2015.

[44] King's College Hospital, 'King's College Hospital and Albany Midwifery Practice', *moderngov.southwark.gov.uk*, 2015.

[45] Lind et al, 2014 in Lokugamage, *The Heart in the Womb*, p.70.

[46] Gaskin, *Spiritual Midwifery*, p.468.

[47] Suzanne in Gaskin, *Spiritual Midwifery*, p.180.

[48] Gaskin, *Ina May's Guide to Childbirth*, p.289.

[49] Russel, 'Could Peripartum Antibiotics have Delayed Health Consequences for the Infant?', *British Journal of Obstetrics and Gynaecology* 113.7, July 2006.

[50] dir. Harman and Wakeford, *Microbirth*, 2014.

[51] Shakespeare, *Romeo and Juliet*, Act 5, Scene 1.

4. MILK

[1] Smillie, 2008, in Mohrbacher and Kendall-Tackett, *Breastfeeding Made Simple: Seven Natural Laws for Nursing Mothers*, p.21.

[2] Gaskin, *Spiritual Midwifery*, p.235.

[3] Colson, 'What Happens to Breastfeeding When Mothers Lie Back? Clinical applications of biological nurturing', *Clinical*

Lactation 1, 2010, p.9.
4   Small, _Our Babies, Ourselves_, p.193.
5   Daly, 'Degree of Breast Emptying Explains Changes in the Fat Content, but Not Fatty Acid Composition, of Human Milk', _Experimental Physiology_ 78.6, 1 November 1993, p.751.
6   Pauline Cross, consultant midwife in Public Health (Lewisham), in conversation with the author, January 2015.
7   Small, _Our Babies, Ourselves_, p.191.
8   Ramsey et al., 'Anatomy of the Lactating Human Breast Redefined with Ultrasound Imaging', _Journal of Anatomy_ 206.6, June 2005.
9   Palmer, _The Politics of Breastfeeding_, p.112.
10 Small, _Our Babies, Ourselves_, p.184.
11 Palmer, _The Politics of Breastfeeding_, p.82.
12 Hopgood, _How Eskimos Keep Their Babies Warm_, p.115.
13 Hopgood, _How Eskimos Keep Their Babies Warm_, p.114.
14 Nestlé UK Ltd., job description for Clinical Network Representative, 14 Apr 2015.
15 Stevens, Patrick and Pickler, 'A History of Infant Feeding', _The Journal of Perinatal Education_ 18.2, Spring 2009.
15 Widdowson, 'Preparations Used for the Artificial Feeding of Infants', _Postgraduate Medical Journal_, March 1978, p.176.
17 Weber et al., 'Lower Protein Content in Infant Formula Reduces BMI and Obesity Risk at School Age: Follow-up of a randomized trial', _The American Journal of Clinical Nutrition_, 12 March 2014.
18 'What's in Breastmilk?', _analyticalarmadillo.co.uk_, 2015.
19 Alkassem et al., 'Structurally Plastic Peptide Capsules for Synthetic Antimicrobial Viruses', _Chemical Science_ 3, 2016.
20 Osborne, 'Breast Milk Drug that "Destroys Cancer" Enters Pre-Clinical Trial Phase', _International Business Times_, 15 October 2013.
21 Lokugamage, _The Heart in the Womb_, p.71; Small, _Our Babies Ourselves_, p.196.
22 Cunningham, 1995, in Small, _Our Babies, Ourselves_, p.196.
23 Baby Milk Action, _babymilkaction.org_, 2015.
24 dir. Wagenhofer, _We Feed the World_, 2005.
25 Palmer, _The Politics of Breastfeeding_, p.230.
26 Palmer, _The Politics of Breastfeeding_, p.228.
27 Baby Milk Action, 'Nestle Targeting Health Workers in the UK',

babymilkaction.org, 2015.

28 Nestlé UK Ltd., job description for Clinical Network Representative,14 April 2015.

29 Jackson, 'Why can't we latch on?', *Guardian*, 11 May 2005.

30 Baby Milk Action, 'How the Nestle Board Excuses Breaking Baby Milk Marketing Rules', *babymilkaction.org*, 2015.

31 Palmer, *The Politics of Breastfeeding*, p.218.

32 *Tigers*, directed by Danis Tanovic and written by Andy Paterson and Danis Tanovic, 2014

33 'Infant Feeding & Early Parenting, Food For Thought...', *analyticalarmadillo.co.uk*, 2016.

34 'Is Iron-Supplementation Necessary?', *kellymom.com*, 2015.

35 Dewey, 'Nutrition, Growth, and Complementary Feeding of the Breastfed Infant', *Pediatric Clinics of North America* 48.1, February 2001.

36 Liedloff, *The Continuum Concept*, p.147.

37 Dettwyler, 'A Time to Wean: The hominid blueprint for the natural age of weaning in modern human populations', *Breastfeeding: Biocultural perspectives*, 1995, p.2.

38 Ochert, 'The Science of Mother's Milk', *New Beginnings* 28.3, 2009, pp.28–29.

39 Dettwyler, 'A Natural Age of Weaning', Department of Anthropology, Texas A and M University, 10 February 2007.

40 Maria Block, in conversation with the author, October 2015.

41 Kamnitzer, 'Breastfeeding in Mongolia', *drmomma.org*, July 2009.

5. SLEEP: SAFE AND SOUND

1 Palmer, *The Politics of Breastfeeding*, p.333.

2 Huffington, 'My Conversation with Co-Sleeping Expert James McKenna', *Huffington Post*, 22 April 2015.

3 Mae, 'Maybe Your Two-Year-Old Just Needs You', *sarahmae.com*, 2013.

4 Small, *Our Babies, Ourselves*, p.99.

5 Small, *Our Babies, Ourselves*, pp.112, 116.

6 Small, *Our Babies, Ourselves*, p.113.

7 Small, *Our Babies, Ourselves*, p.222.

8 Liedloff, *The Continuum Concept*, p.75.

9   Ferber, *Solve Your Child's Sleep Problems*, p.40.

10 Ferber, *Solve Your Child's Sleep Problems*, p.41.

11 Small, *Our Babies, Ourselves*, p.113.

12 McKenna, 'Night Waking among Breastfeeding Mothers and Infants: Conflict, congruence or both?', *Evolution, Medicine, and Public Health*, 2014, p.43.

13 Liedloff, *The Continuum Concept*, p.31.

14 Small, *Our Babies, Ourselves*, p.117.

15 Hegarty, 'The Myth of the Eight-Hour Sleep', *BBC Magazine*, 22 February 2012.

16 Hegarty, 'The Myth of the Eight-Hour Sleep', *BBC Magazine*, 22 February 2012.

17 Hegarty, 'The Myth of the Eight-Hour Sleep', *BBC Magazine*, 22 February 2012.

18 McKenna, 'Dr. McKenna's Biography', *cosleeping.nd.edu/mckenna-biography*, 2016.

19 Bergman, 'Bed Sharing Per Se Is Not Dangerous', *JAMA Pediatrics* 167.11, November 2013, pp.998–99.

20 McKenna, Ball and Gettler, 'Mother–Infant Cosleeping, Breastfeeding and Sudden Infant Death Syndrome', *Yearbook of Physical Anthropology* 134.S45, 2007. pp.133–61.

21 Huffington, 'My Conversation with Co-Sleeping Expert James McKenna', *Huffington Post*, 22 April 2015.

22 McKenna, 'Cosleeping and Biological Imperatives: Why human babies do not and should not sleep alone', *neuroanthropology.net*, 21 December 2008.

23 McKenna, Ball and Gettler, 'Mother–Infant Cosleeping, Breastfeeding and Sudden Infant Death Syndrome', *Yearbook of Physical Anthropology* 50, 2007, p.147.

24 McKenna, Ball and Gettler, 'Mother–Infant Cosleeping, Breastfeeding and Sudden Infant Death Syndrome', *Yearbook of Physical Anthropology* 50, 2007, p.149.

25 Small, *Our Babies, Ourselves*, p.129.

26 Small, *Our Babies, Ourselves*, p.122.

27 Gettler et al., 'Does Cosleeping Contribute to Lower Testosterone Levels in Fathers? Evidence from the Philippines', *plos.org*, 5 September 2012.

28 Rapaport, 'Mad Women and Desperate Girls: Infanticide and child murder in law and myth', *Fordham Urban Law Journal* 33.2, 2005, p.122.

29 Small, *Our Babies, Ourselves*, p.122.

30 Small, *Our Babies, Ourselves*, p.82.

31 McKenna, Ball and Gettler, 'Mother–Infant Cosleeping, Breastfeeding and Sudden Infant Death Syndrome', *Yearbook of Physical Anthropology* 50, 2007, p.143.

32 Huffington, 'My Conversation with Co-Sleeping Expert James McKenna', *Huffington Post*, 22 April 2015.

33 Ferber, *How to Solve Your Child's Sleep Problems*, pp.180–83.

34 Ferber, 'Sleeping with the Baby', *New Yorker*, 8 November 1999.

35 Gerhardt, *Why Love Matters*, p.10.

36 Gerhardt, *Why Love Matters*, p.37.

37 O'Doherty et al., 'Dissociating Valence of Outcome from Behavioral Control in Human Orbital and Ventral Prefrontal Cortices', *The Journal of Neuroscience*, 27 August 2003, p.7,939.

38 Gerhardt, *Why Love Matters*, p.38.

39 Gerhardt, *Why Love Matters*, p.91.

40 Gerhardt, *Why Love Matters*, p.175.

41 Steingard et al., 'Smaller Frontal Lobe White Matter Volumes in Depressed Adolescents', *Biological Psychiatry* 52.5, 1 September 2002, pp.413–17.

42 Gerhardt, *Why Love Matters*, p.126.

43 Gerhardt, *Why Love Matters*, p.126.

44 Gerhardt, *Why Love Matters*, p.91.

45 McEwen, 'Allostasis and Allostatic Load: Implications for neuropsychopharmacology', *Neuropsychopharmacology* 22.2, February 2000, pp.108–24.

46 Gerhardt, *Why Love Matters*, p.64.

47 Gerhardt, *Why Love Matters*, p.127.

48 Lewis and Janda, 'The Relationship Between Adult Sexual Adjustment and Childhood Experience Regarding Exposure to Nudity, Sleeping in the Parental Bed, and Parental Attitudes Toward Sexuality', *Archives of Sexual Behaviour* 17, 1988, pp.349–62.

49 Crawford, 'Parenting Practices in the Basque Country: Implications of infant and childhood sleeping location for

personality development', *Ethos: Journal of the Society for Psychological Anthropology* 22.1, March 1994, pp.42–82.

50 Heron, *Nonreactive Co-sleeping and Child Behavior: Getting a Good Night's Sleep All Night Every Night*, Masters Thesis, University of Bristol, 1994.

51 McCaleb in Interview with Bevan, 'How to Nurture Your Child's Brain Development in the Early Years', *The Confident Mother*, 2015, p.11–12.

52 Anders, 'Self-Soothing: Possibly biggest lie ever foisted on parents', *uncommonjohn.wordpress.com*, 4 January 2013; 'The Researcher Who Helped Coin the Term Self-Soothing Weighs In', *uncommonjohn.wordpress.com*, 27 September 2014.

6. STRONG FOUNDATIONS

1   Grille, *Parenting for a Peaceful World*, p.101.
2   Nicholson and Parker, *Attached at the Heart*, p.5.
3   Anan in, Grille, *Parenting for a Peaceful World*, p.1.
4   Odent, 'The First Hour Following Birth: Don't wake the mother!', *Midwifery Today*, 61, Spring 2002, p.9–11.
5   Grille, *Parenting for a Peaceful World*, p.5.
6   Grille, *Parenting for a Peaceful World*, pp.7, 104.
7   Bowlby, *A Secure Base*, pp.38–39.
8   Bowlby, *A Secure Base*, p.55.
9   Liedloff, *The Continuum Concept*, p.87.
10 Bowlby, *A Secure Base*, p.51.
11 Gerhardt, *Why Love Matters*, p.72.
12 Gerhardt, *Why Love Matters*, p.65.
13 Hopgood, *How Eskimos Keep Their Babies Warm*, p.11.
14 Hopgood, *How Eskimos Keep Their Babies Warm*, p.10.
15 Bowlby, *A Secure Base*, p.17.
16 Hewlett, 'Multiple Caretaking among African Pygmies', *American Anthropologist* 91.1, March 1989, pp.186–91.
17 Small, *Our Babies, Ourselves*, p.25.
18 Liedloff, *The Continuum Concept*, p.139.
19 Liedloff, *The Continuum Concept*, p.14.
20 Bowlby, *A Secure Base*, p.2.
21 Hopgood, *How Eskimos Keep their Babies Warm*, p.196.

22 van de Rijt and Plooij, *The Wonder Weeks*, p.36.
23 Candiano-Marcus, *Baby Prodigy: A Guide to Raising a Smarter, Happier Baby*, p.108.
24 Biggs, 'The "Epidemic" of Deformational Plagiocephaly and the American Academy of Pediatrics' Response', *Journal of Prosthetics and Orthotics* 16, 2004, pp.5–8.
25 Hopgood, *How Eskimos Keep Their Babies Warm*, p.69.
26 Biggs, 'The "Epidemic" of Deformational Plagiocephaly and the American Academy of Pediatrics' Response', *Journal of Prosthetics and Orthotics* 16, 2004, pp.5–8.
27 Hobbs, 'The "Container Baby" Lifestyle', *North Shore Pediatric Therapy*, 4 May 2011.
28 Harkness and Super, 1992; Harkness et al., 2009; Super, 1983.
29 Gaskin, *Spiritual Midwifery*, p.242.
30 van de Rijt and Plooij, *The Wonder Weeks*, p.31.
31 Bowlby, *A Secure Base*, p.10.
32 Bowlby, *A Secure Base*, p.10.
33 Liedloff, *The Continuum Concept*, p.24
34 Gerhardt, *Why Love Matters*, p.191.

7. TWO STEPS FORWARD, ONE STEP BACK

1 van de Rijt and Plooij, *The Wonder Weeks*, pp.15, 42.
2 van de Rijt and Plooij, *The Wonder Weeks*, p.2.
3 van de Rijt and Plooij, *The Wonder Weeks*, p.444.
4 van de Rijt and Plooij, *The Wonder Weeks*, p.41.
5 van de Rijt and Plooij, *The Wonder Weeks*, p.80.
6 van de Rijt and Plooij, *The Wonder Weeks*, p.13.
7 van de Rijt and Plooij, *The Wonder Weeks*, p.46.
8 van de Rijt and Plooij, *The Wonder Weeks*, p.46.
9 van de Rijt and Plooij, *The Wonder Weeks*, p.443.

8. TOTALLY POTTY

1 Anonymous, *Don'ts for Mothers*, 1878, republished 2011.
2 Hatch, *Nappy Free Baby*, p.21.
3 Hatch, *Nappy Free Baby*, p.29.
4 Hatch, *Nappy Free Baby*, p.64.
5 Backaler, 'How Procter & Gamble Cultivates Customers in

China', *Forbes*, 27 April 2010.

[6] Hopgood, *How Eskimos Keep Their Babies Warm*, p.83.

[7] Hopgood, *How Eskimos Keep Their Babies Warm*, p.87.

[8] Boucke, *Infant Potty Training*, p.318.

[9] Hatch, *Nappy Free Baby*, p.135.

[10] Hatch, *Nappy Free Baby*, p.131.

[11] Hatch, *Nappy Free Baby*, p.231.

9. LOVE IS THE LAW

[1] Liedloff, *The Continuum Concept*, p.35.

SELECTED BIBLIOGRAPHY

Boucke, Laurie, *Infant Potty Training* (White-Boucke: 2008)

Bowlby, John, *A Secure Base* (Routledge: 2012)

Candiano-Marcus, Barbara, *Baby Prodigy* (Random House: 2009)

Enright, Anne, *Making Babies* (Cape: 2004)

Ferber, Richard, *Solve Your Child's Sleep Problems* (DK: 1986)

Gaskin, Ina May, *Birth Matters* (Pinter & Martin: 2011)

Gaskin, Ina May, *Ina May's Guide to Childbirth* (Vermilion: 2008)

Gaskin, Ina May, *Spiritual Midwifery* (Book Publishing Company: 2010)

Gerhardt, Sue, *Why Love Matters* (Taylor & Francis: 2004)

Grille, Robin, *Parenting for a Peaceful World* (CP Publishing: 2008)

Hatch, Amber, *Nappy Free Baby* (Random House: 2015)

Hopgood, Mei Ling, *How Eskimos Keep Their Babies Warm* (Algonquin Books: 2012)

Liedloff, Jean, *The Continuum Concept* (Penguin: 2004)

Lokugamage, Amali, *The Heart in the Womb* (Docamali: 2011)

Mohrbacher, Nancy and Kendall-Tackett, Kathleen, *Breastfeeding Made Simple: Seven Natural Laws for Nursing Mothers* (New Harbinger Publications: 2010)

Nicholson, Barbara and Parker, Lysa, *Attached at the Heart* (Health Communications: 2013)

Palmer, *The Politics of Breastfeeding,* 3rd edition (Pinter & Martin: 2009)

Small, Meredith, *Our Babies, Ourselves* (Knopf Doubleday: 2011)

Stone, Lawrence, *The Family, Sex and Marriage in England 1500–1800* (Weidenfeld & Nicolson: 1977)

van de Rijt, Hetty and Plooij, Frans X. *The Wonder Weeks* (Kiddy World Promotions: 2010)

Wertz, Richard W. and Wertz, Dorothy C., *Lying-in: A History of Childbirth in America* (Yale University Press: 1989)

FILMOGRAPHY

Harman, Toni and Wakeford, Alex, *Freedom for Birth* (UK, 2012)

Pascale-Bonaro, Debra, *Orgasmic Birth* (USA, 2009)

Harman, Toni and Wakeford, Alex, *Microbirth* (UK, 2014)

Wagenhofer, Erwin, *We Feed the World* (Austria, 2005)

INDEX